Thee Chronic Illness Exit Plan

by

Dr June Williams DMedEth

The Chronic Illness Exit Plan - First Edition

Table of contents

1. Acknowledgements 5
2. Disclaimer 6
3. Foreword 7
4. Chapter One - When "Normal" Doesn't Feel Normal 19
5. Chapter Two - When Trying Harder Makes It Worse 33
6. Chapter Three - When Treatments That Should Work Don't 61
7. Chapter Four - When Talking Can Make the Body Worse 95
8. Chapter Five - Clearing the Fog - Why Your Brain Is Not Broken 126
9. Chapter Six - Rebuilding Trust - With Your Body and the Future 160
10. Afterword 197

Acknowledgements

The clinical examples and personal stories in this book are shared with informed consent. All identifying details have been changed, and in some cases elements have been combined, to protect privacy while preserving the integrity of the experiences described.

My sincere thanks to those who entrusted me with their journeys. Your openness has contributed to a clearer, more compassionate understanding of chronic illness—one that I hope will help others feel less alone and more understood.

Disclaimer

This book has not been evaluated by any medical or regulatory authority. It is provided for informational and educational purposes only and is not intended to diagnose, treat, prevent, or cure any disease or medical condition.

The content should not be considered medical advice or a substitute for consultation with a qualified healthcare professional. Readers are responsible for seeking appropriate professional guidance regarding their own health decisions.

The author and publisher make no representations regarding the accuracy or suitability of the information provided and accept no liability for any outcomes resulting from its use. All views and opinions expressed are those of the author and do not necessarily reflect those of any other individual or organisation.

Foreword

It's 3:17 a.m.

You're awake again.

Not properly awake. Not properly asleep. Just stuck in that grey in-between where your body won't rest and your mind is too tired to think clearly.

The house is quiet. The fridge hums. The clock ticks. Loudly.

You've meant to move that clock. For months. But standing up, bending down, reaching behind the table feels absurdly demanding. Not dramatic. Just too much.

That's the part that's hard to explain to anyone.

Your head feels thick. Like cotton wool. Your jaw is tight. Your heart isn't racing, but it isn't settled either. Just alert enough to keep you here.

You turn over.

That dull resistance blooms in your joints. Not sharp pain. Not something that makes you cry out. Just the familiar background ache. The one that never really leaves.

You negotiate with it.

If I move slowly.
If I don't twist.
If I breathe carefully.

Do you remember when moving didn't require strategy?

Your phone lights up. An article you saved weeks ago stares back at you: what to do when your tests are normal but you still feel terrible.

You don't open it.

You already know what it says.

Manage stress. Improve sleep. Gentle exercise. Magnesium. Therapy. Acceptance.

The truth is... you've tried.

You have another appointment tomorrow.

Another professional who will glance at your results and say, "Everything looks fine... Stable... within range”

And this is the hard truth.

When nothing is wrong on paper, something starts to feel wrong with you.

You rehearse your answers in your head.

Yes, you’ve tried that.
Yes, you eat well.
Yes, you’ve exercised when you can.
No, you’re not depressed. You’re exhausted.

There’s a particular loneliness to this kind of illness.

You look fine. You function enough. You cancel plans quietly. You rest without feeling restored. You adapt without improving.

And somewhere in the dark, you remember who you used to be.

Not superhuman. Just available. You had spare energy. You made plans without calculating the cost.

Now everything is calculated.

You're not asking for a miracle. You'd settle for reliable.

And beneath it all sits the question you don't say out loud:

Is this it?

When I went through my own version of this, that question terrified me more than any symptom. Not the pain. Not the fatigue. The shrinking.

The truth is… no one tells you how frightening slow decline feels when it isn't dramatic enough to justify panic.

You lie there waiting for morning.

Hoping someone, somewhere, has missed something.

Let me say something clearly.

Your body is not broken.

The truth is... it is overwhelmed.

That's different.

Modern medicine is exceptional at finding damage. Tumours. Infections. Fractures. Severe inflammation. If something is structurally wrong, we are very good at spotting it.

But here's the uncomfortable reality.

You can feel dreadful long before anything looks dramatic on a scan.

Really, this is what I've found over and over again. In research. In clinic. In my own life.

Tests measure damage. They do not measure regulation.

You can have numbers "within range" and still have a system that is struggling to coordinate itself.

Think of an orchestra. Every instrument intact. Every musician trained. But no conductor. Timing lost. Sound becomes noise.

Nothing is broken. But nothing is coherent either.

That's what chronic dysregulation feels like.

When I was working in pharmaceutical research, I saw this gap repeatedly. We could measure pathology with precision. But the grey zone? The space where people were suffering without structural failure? That space was uncomfortable.

So it often became psychological.

Stress. Coping. Perception.

Now let's be honest. Stress absolutely affects the body. Of course it does. But stress is not a character flaw.

And the truth is... telling someone to "manage stress" when their nervous system is already exhausted can feel like blame dressed as advice.

Here is what is often happening instead.

Your system has been in subtle defence for too long.

Not emergency panic. Not collapse. Just a low, steady state of bracing.

Sleep becomes lighter. Muscles stay guarded. Digestion becomes inconsistent. Energy gets diverted toward vigilance instead of repair.

You keep going. But the bandwidth narrows.

When I say "regulation precedes recovery," I mean this: you cannot optimise a body that feels unsafe.

You can add supplements. You can gain insight. You can eat beautifully. You can exercise with discipline.

But if the underlying state is defensive, the gains won't stick.

Really, this is what I've found.

People don't fail protocols. Protocols fail depleted systems.

That's a hard truth.

It's not about motivation. It's not about belief.

It's not about how positive you are.

It's about load.

Too many signals. Not enough resolution.

And when the system is overloaded, even good interventions can feel like more input.

The answer is not to try harder.

The truth is... it's often to reduce.

Reduce noise. Reduce interference. Reduce unnecessary activation.

When the body feels less threatened, it reorganises itself. Not magically. Biologically.

Your symptoms may have started as protection. The problem is when protection never switches off.

And until that softens, nothing truly integrates.

Now imagine something simple.

You wake up and your body feels quieter.

Not perfect. Not euphoric. Just less loud.

Your thoughts come online without that cotton-wool thickness. You stand up without bracing. You make a plan without calculating collapse.

What would that change?

When regulation begins to return, it's subtle at first.

Sleep deepens. Not longer. Deeper.

Digestion steadies. Mood feels proportionate. You are less startled by ordinary life.

You stop chasing every new protocol because you can feel what helps and what doesn't.

And here's something important.

You begin to trust your own feedback again.

When I experienced that shift myself, it wasn't fireworks. It was relief. Quiet relief.

The truth is... safety in the body feels boring.

And boring is beautiful when you've lived in constant alert.

You no longer live as if one wrong decision will undo everything.

That's freedom.

Not symptom-free perfection. But capacity.

Capacity to adapt. To recover. To expand again.

Really, this is what matters most.

Not erasing every sensation. Restoring resilience.

So where does this begin?

Not with force.

Not with belief.

Not with pushing through.

It begins with a sequence.

The Body Reset Framework™ is built on a simple principle: reduce interference before adding intensity.

You will explore why chronic symptoms are often better understood as signal overload rather than damage. You will see how nervous system safety influences everything else. You will understand why trying harder has likely made things worse.

And that's not a criticism.

It's biology.

You will not be asked to relive trauma. You will not be asked to adopt heroic routines.

You will be guided to observe.

To notice.

To remove what keeps the system braced.

The exit is not dramatic.

The truth is... it feels more like early spring.

At first, you barely notice the thaw.

Then one day you realise you are not calculating every movement anymore.

You are not broken.

You are overloaded.

And really, this is what I've found time and again—

When interference decreases, regulation returns.

Not instantly.

But reliably.

And that is where we begin.

Chapter One - When "Normal" Doesn't Feel Normal

You sit in a consultation room.

The screen glows. The clinician scrolls.

They smile kindly and say,
"There's nothing here that explains how bad you feel."

It sounds like good news.

So why does it land like a loss?

You nod. You thank them. You walk out carrying the same exhausted body you walked in with.

Only now you're carrying something else.

Doubt.

The blood tests are normal.
The scan is clear.
The ECG is fine.

And yet your heart still races. Your joints still ache. Your sleep still collapses at 3am. You still wake tired.

So what are you supposed to do with that?

Here is the uncomfortable truth: when you're told you're fine but you don't feel fine, something fractures.

At first, you question the system.
Then you question yourself.

Are you overreacting?
Are you just stressed?
Are you not coping well enough?

What became unmistakably clear to me over years in research and practice is this: the moment you start doubting your own experience is the moment you start pushing harder.

You research more.
You tighten your diet.
You add supplements.
You optimise.

Because if nothing is wrong, then maybe you

just need to try harder.

But biology does not reward pressure.

And the nervous system operates on rules, not willpower.

Trying harder is often what destabilises a system already on edge.

Across case after case, one pattern kept emerging.

A woman came to see me after having multiple cardiac stents fitted. Structurally, her heart had been repaired. The cardiology reports were balanced. The team were satisfied.

On paper, everything was stable.

Yet she still had episodes of tachycardia. Sudden racing pulse. Emotional swings. A body that wouldn't settle.

When I first met her, she said, "But they fixed it."

Yes. They fixed the structure.

But no one had addressed the state.

When we shifted attention toward calming her nervous system rather than pursuing more mechanical intervention, her episodes reduced. Not magically. Not theatrically. But measurably.

Over time, a consistent thread revealed itself:

Normal tests do not automatically mean a regulated system.

Structure and regulation are not the same thing.

Medicine is exceptional at detecting damage.
It is less equipped to detect instability.

And instability is what you feel.

Signal Reception Theory™

At some point, you have to ask a different question.

Not, “What else can I take?”

But, “Can my body actually receive anything right now?”

This is where Signal Reception Theory™ shifts the lens.

Most chronically unwell bodies are not broken.

They are overloaded.

There is a difference.

A body has to be able to receive before it can respond.

You take magnesium to calm your system. Instead, you feel foggy.
You try a supplement that helped someone else. Your heart races.
You follow a carefully designed protocol. You crash harder.

Why?

Because an overloaded nervous system reads input as demand.

It does not distinguish between helpful and harmful. It recognises more.

And when you have been in survival mode for

months or years, more feels unsafe.

If I strip this back to first principles, the pattern is simple:

If the system is saturated, even the correct intervention lands like pressure.

The woman with cardiac stents did not need stronger intervention.

She needed sequencing.

Mechanically repaired.
Functionally dysregulated.

When emotional threat softened, tachycardia softened.

The receiver changed.

The intervention did not.

Timing Over Dosage

We have been trained to think in terms of dose.

If 200 mg doesn't work, try 400.
If one session doesn't help, book six.
If fatigue continues, escalate.

But what if the issue isn't quantity?

What if it is timing?

The body works in rhythms. Protection phases. Repair phases.

If you introduce something before the system feels safe enough to receive it, it will defend.

And defence looks like symptom flare.

Not failure.
Not weakness.
Timing.

Cells respond to safety before they respond to chemistry.

That principle alone changes everything.

Signal Clarity Over Intensity

How many things are you doing right now in the name of getting better?

Morning supplements.
Special diets.
Evening minerals.
Tracking apps.
Breathing protocols.
Advice from five directions.

Each makes sense alone.

Together? Noise.

Imagine ten people speaking to you at once.

At some point, you stop listening.

The nervous system is no different.

When signals stack, clarity drops.

Receptors dampen responsiveness.

And then you say, “Nothing works anymore.”

But the signal has been buried under layering.

I have watched clients pause almost everything. No drama. Just subtraction.

Symptoms did not vanish overnight.

But they softened.

Sleep steadied.
Heart rhythm became less reactive.
Energy crashes lost intensity.

Weeks later, an intervention that previously failed was reintroduced at half the dose.

This time, it worked.

The supplement had not changed.

The receiver had.

The Hard Truth — and the Relief

Let's be honest about this.

Your body is not failing you.

It is protecting you.

Chronic symptoms often reflect a system processing too much for too long without sufficient safety.

Not broken.

Overloaded.

Laboratory ranges are statistical averages. They tell you whether you sit inside a population band.

They do not tell you whether your nervous system feels safe.

You can be inside range and outside balance.

Like a house standing upright while the wiring flickers behind the walls.

You feel the flicker long before anyone sees

smoke.

The absence of visible damage does not equal the presence of harmony.

That is not mystical.

It is physiological.

This Week: Stop Fixing

You have tried hard.

So this week, you do something different.

You stop fixing.

You start observing.

Take a notebook. Real paper.

Write down symptoms as they occur.

Not interpretation.
Not meaning.
Not Google.

Just data.

"Heart racing at 3pm."
"Exhausted after supermarket."
"Jaw tight on waking."

When you remove narrative, patterns surface.

A permanently damaged structure does not fluctuate.

A dysregulated system does.

Circle what fluctuates.

Underline what eases.

Ask yourself:

Does this look broken?
Or reactive?

Pause one non-essential add-on this week.

Not medication.
Not medical instruction.

One layer of noise.

And observe.

You are not giving up.

You are reducing interference.

The Shift

Here is what became clear long before I opened a clinic:

The problem is systemic, not personal.

You were never failing treatment.

Treatment failed sequencing.

That distinction restores agency.

You are not weak.
You are not dramatic.
You are not defective.

You are a living system that has been bracing.

Once you understand that symptoms can signal

disorganisation rather than defect, something steadies.

Clarity restores influence.

And when you stop seeing yourself as broken, you can finally see what is actually happening.

In the next chapter, we explore something many resist hearing at first:

Why trying harder may be amplifying the instability you want to escape.

Because a system in defence does not respond well to pressure.

It responds to safety.

And that is where we turn next.

Chapter Two - When Trying Harder Makes It Worse

You sit in the consultation room while the clinician scrolls through your results.

They are kind. Professional. Calm.

Then it comes.

“There’s nothing here that explains how bad you feel.”

You smile politely. You nod. You leave.

But you walk out carrying something new alongside the symptoms.

Doubt.

That sentence lands harder than anyone realises.

Because if nothing explains how you feel, what does that make you? Over-sensitive? Anxious? Dramatic? Failing at coping?

Being told you are "fine" when you are not doesn't just confuse you. It fractures trust. First in medicine. Then in yourself.

And once that crack appears, something subtle happens.

You try harder.

You clean up your diet again. You research more. You add supplements. You remove supplements. You track your sleep. You monitor your steps. You meditate properly this time. You do the breathing correctly. You become disciplined.

Hyper-responsible.

But let me ask you something gently.

What if trying harder is part of why you are more tired?

When tests rule out disease, they often rule out damage. They do not rule out strain. They do not measure nervous system overload. They do not measure energy depletion. They do not measure how long you've been compensating.

And compensation is exhausting.

I once worked with a woman who had lived her whole life with an extremely rare condition. Monitored. Managed. Supervised. She was medically brilliant about her own body. Exceptionally compliant.

But when I asked her to tell me about herself, she didn't talk about what she loved. She didn't talk about her personality. She didn't even talk about her life.

She talked about her diagnosis.

That was who she had become.

When I saw that, it stopped me.

Because really this is what I've found: long-term illness can quietly replace your identity. You become the syndrome. The case. The file.

Before we did anything to "treat" her body, we did something else.

We helped her remember who she was.

For years she had done everything right. She followed the guidance. Took the medication. Attended the appointments. Improved on paper.

And then, despite all of that effort, she suffered an embolism.

Collapse after compliance.

That moment was sobering. For her. For me.

Because it showed us something uncomfortable.

Stability had been maintained by constant effort. Not by deep resilience.

Borrowed strength is not the same as true regulation.

And I have seen this pattern more times than I can count. When I worked inside systems that valued control and optimisation above all else, I watched how people could look "stable" while quietly running on fumes. When I pushed harder in my own life, determined to override what my body was signalling, I paid for it later.

You cannot bully a nervous system into safety.

So let me ask you something honestly.

Have you become more disciplined... or more afraid?

Are you improving... or just managing better?

There's a hard truth here.

If you have been living in survival mode for years, more effort feels like more threat. Even if it looks like virtue.

You wake already calculating. How much can I do today? What will trigger a crash? How carefully must I live?

That is not weakness. That is adaptation.

And adaptation has a cost.

With that same woman, our early sessions were not technical. No clever interventions. No dramatic protocols.

We focused on something deceptively simple.

Helping her feel real again.

Not a patient. Not a syndrome. A person.

As that shifted, her symptoms softened. Not instantly. Not magically. But steadily. Her body stopped gripping quite so tightly. Regulation followed safety.

Systems stabilise when the person inside them feels recognised.

So when a clinician tells you nothing explains how bad you feel, the danger is not just dismissal.

The danger is that you internalise it.

You decide the problem must be you.

And then you try harder.

But really this is what I've found after decades inside medicine and outside it: chronic strain is rarely solved by more discipline. It is resolved by understanding what the body has been compensating for.

Before we ask how you can manage better, we need a different question.

What has your system been carrying alone?

That question changes the direction of everything.

The Effort–Capacity Mismatch™

In the opening of this chapter, you met the woman who did everything right.

She complied.
She monitored.
She endured.

She became admirable in her discipline.

And yet her system collapsed.

That is not a dramatic anecdote. It is the logical outcome of what happens when effort exceeds capacity for too long.

Trying harder can make you worse.

Not because effort is bad.
But because effort has a cost.

Let's return to her for a moment—not as a

separate story, but as a mirror.

When she first came to see me, she did not introduce herself as a person.

She introduced herself as a condition.

Decades of living with an extremely rare diagnosis had quietly reshaped her identity. She described lab trends, medication tolerances, specialist opinions. She spoke in data. She had become fluent in survival.

But somewhere along the way, she had disappeared.

When you become your syndrome, the nervous system never truly stands down. It is always guarding. Always measuring. Always braced.

Before we touched her physiology, we had to retrieve her.

Because if your entire existence revolves around managing symptoms, even your good days become transactions. You do not enjoy them. You extract from them.

You wake clearer and think, Quick. Use this.

And then you crash.

Does that sound familiar?

This is Step One of the Effort–Capacity Mismatch™: Borrowed Energy.

On her "good" days, she would over-function. She had been trained to maximise every window of stability. That is what responsible patients do.

But those windows were not true strength.

They were stress-supported surges.

The body can temporarily override fragility. Adrenaline sharpens the mind. Cortisol mobilises fuel. You can look stable. You can feel capable.

I have done this myself in earlier in my life. When I was working in high-pressure environments, I could function brilliantly on drive alone. I mistook output for health.

But the bill always came.

Activation is not repair.

When you are depleted, pushing on a good day often means you are spending tomorrow's resources today.

And the crash is not failure.

It is accounting.

In her case, the deeper cost did not show immediately. For years she complied perfectly. Careful supervision. Regular monitoring. Structured living. From the outside, she was stable.

Then she suffered an embolism.

Out of nowhere, it seemed.

But it was not nowhere.

It was the exposure of borrowed stability.

Despite doing everything correctly, her system had never rebuilt true capacity. It had been held together by vigilance and effort.

And here is the hard truth: you can look stable

while being fragile.

Management can create the appearance of control. It does not always create resilience.

Which brings us to Step Two: Management Fatigue.

Have you noticed how much mental energy you spend managing yourself?

Every decision filtered through symptoms.
Every invitation evaluated.
Every meal analysed.
Every sensation interpreted.

You are not just living.

You are supervising.

And supervision is effort.

The woman I'm describing had reached a point where her entire life was structured around preventing deterioration. Even her thoughts were clinical. Even her language was medical.

When collapse came, it was not because she was

careless.

It was because her system had never experienced true downshift.

Regulation grows in safety, not in surveillance.

The body does not rebuild strength under constant watchfulness. It rebuilds when it feels secure enough to allocate resources to repair.

So we did something that initially felt almost irresponsible.

We subtracted.

That is Step Three.

We removed certain layers of monitoring that had become compulsive rather than helpful. We stopped chasing micro-adjustments. We simplified her routines.

But more importantly, we retrieved her.

We talked about who she had been before the diagnosis. What she enjoyed. What she believed about herself. What she missed.

Because systems stabilise when the person feels real again.

And slowly, as her identity widened beyond illness, her symptoms softened. Sleep deepened. Pain flares shortened. Emotional volatility reduced.

No dramatic breakthrough.

Just steadiness.

That steadiness did not come from trying harder.

It came from reducing load.

The Effort–Capacity Mismatch™ is simple, but confronting.

If your daily management requires more energy than your body can spare, you are perpetuating instability.

And you will feel confused.

You will say, But I'm doing everything right.

Yes.

That may be exactly the problem.

Trying harder is seductive. It feels active. Responsible. Strong.

Subtraction feels passive. Almost lazy.

But the truth is... when capacity is low, effort becomes extraction.

And extraction leads to collapse.

You do not rebuild a burned forest by running through it with fertiliser. You protect the soil. You reduce disturbance. You allow rhythm to return.

So let me ask you something gently.

Where are you still extracting from yourself in the name of improvement?

Where are you squeezing productivity out of "good days" that were meant for restoration?

And what would change if your goal was not to maximise function—but to stabilise capacity?

When effort finally matches available energy,

the oscillation between surge and crash begins to narrow.

The drama reduces.

The fear softens.

And the body—quietly, almost imperceptibly—starts to trust again.

Not because you fought harder.

But because you finally stopped asking it to prove itself.

We have been exploring a difficult idea.

That effort, when it becomes your identity, can quietly destabilise you.

That compliance is not the same as safety.
That management is not the same as resilience.

Now we bring that down to ground level. Into your actual day.

Because this is not abstract. It is lived.

And really, this is what I've found after years of practice: the people who try the hardest are often the ones who are most exhausted.

Start here.

Take a pen and write down everything you are currently managing.

Not just treatments. Everything.

- Supplements.
- Food rules.
- Sleep routines.
- Tracking apps.
- Specialist appointments.
- The quiet calculations you make before agreeing to anything.

Be honest.

How much of your mental bandwidth is devoted to preventing decline?

When I did this exercise myself years ago, I expected to feel organised. Instead, I felt tense. I realised I was never off duty.

And the truth is... the nervous system does not relax when it is permanently supervising.

One woman I worked with had lived for decades with a rare condition. When I asked her to describe herself, she didn't tell me about her character or her passions.

She told me her diagnosis.

She had slowly become her syndrome.

It wasn't dramatic. It was incremental. Years of monitoring had replaced identity with management. Every decision filtered through symptoms. Every conversation framed by risk.

Before we addressed her physiology, we had to ask a more fundamental question.

Who are you beneath this?

Recovery began not with intervention, but with remembering.

When the person reappears, the system begins to settle.

There is a harder truth.

This same woman did everything correctly.

She complied. She attended. She followed every instruction carefully. On paper, she looked stable.

Then she had an embolism.

It felt sudden. Shocking. Unfair.

But when we stepped back, the pattern was visible. Her stability had been held together by constant effort. It had not become internally robust. It was managed stability. Borrowed resilience.

And the truth is... you can be diligent and still fragile.

Effort can mask depletion.

That is not blame. It is biology.

So what do you do?

You subtract.

Choose one layer of management and remove it for seven days.

Not recklessly. Thoughtfully.

Perhaps it is the nightly symptom scoring.
Perhaps it is the third supplement added "just in case."
Perhaps it is an online community that keeps you immersed in illness language.

Ask yourself a simple question: does this create safety, or does it reinforce vigilance?

Be careful not to replace it with something else. This is the subtle trap. Swapping strict control for gentle control. Replacing one tracking system with another that feels more holistic but carries the same demand.

The pattern is the problem.

Cancel one tracking habit entirely.

Delete the app.

Stop rating your fatigue.

Notice what happens.

When I guide people through this, they expect chaos. Often what they feel instead is space. A small but real exhale.

Constant monitoring keeps the body braced.

Simplify your meals.

For one week, choose three nourishing, familiar meals and rotate them. Remove performance. Remove experimentation.

Food has likely become strategic. Evaluated. Controlled.

Let it become ordinary.

Ordinary is regulating.

And then, the most uncomfortable step.

Rest without purpose.

Not to recover faster.
Not to improve metrics.
Not to optimise.

Just rest.

When I first practised purposeless rest, I felt restless. Irritated. I realised how deeply I equated effort with worth.

Many of you fear stopping more than you fear symptoms.

But the body cannot shift out of survival while you are constantly proving you are trying.

In early sessions with that same woman, we spent time not on treatment, but on reclamation.

We talked about who she had been before illness took centre stage.

Her interests.
Her humour.
Her unfinished ambitions.

As she began to feel like a person again, her symptoms softened. Not dramatically. Not magically. But steadily.

Regulation followed recognition.

Systems stabilise when the person feels real again.

There are three common mistakes here.

1. Mistaking rest for laziness.
2. Adding "just one gentle thing."
3. Replacing one rigid system with another dressed in new language.

You do not need more optimisation. You need less demand.

So here is your quick win.

Today, do nothing extra.

No new supplement.
No new research.
No new adjustment.

Let the day be enough.

And notice.

Does something in you soften?

You are not broken.

You are over-managing.

When effort loosens, safety has space to return.

That is where real resilience begins.

You have tried harder than most people will ever know.

You tried to follow every instruction.
You tried to be compliant.
You tried to stay hopeful.

You changed your diet. Added supplements. Took the medication. Read the books. Sat in the therapy chair. Joined the forums. Did the breathing exercises. Rested when told. Pushed when told.

And when nothing truly shifted, what did you conclude?

That you weren't doing enough.

You were doing too much inside a system that didn't feel safe.

Really, this is what I've found after decades inside both clinical research and lived illness: when the body does not respond, it is not refusing. It is protecting.

Non-response is a signal, not a verdict.

But no one tells you that.

Instead, the subtle message becomes: try harder. Be more disciplined. Be more positive. Find the right practitioner. The right protocol. The right mindset.

Let me ask you something.

If effort alone fixed this, wouldn't you be well by now?

Treatments fail when reception is impaired. Not because they are useless. Not because you are broken. But because your system cannot safely receive what is being offered.

Timing determines outcome more than dosage.

You can give the "right" thing at the wrong time and the body will tighten instead of soften.

I learned this the hard way.

When I was sitting in that meeting and the angioedema began—itching, swelling, the familiar warning—I could feel my system bracing. I had braced for years. Braced in consultations. Braced in corridors. Braced while being spoken over.

And when I finally stopped shrinking... when I paused the call and said, "I will not continue without proper representation"... something shifted.

The swelling receded.

No new drug. No higher dose. Just clarity.

And really, this is what I've found: clarity restores cooperation.

The body relaxes when the internal conflict stops.

You were not resistant to healing.

Read that again.

You were not resistant.

Your system was protecting itself from

overload.

Every time you pushed through fatigue.
Every time you overrode your own hesitation.
Every time you told yourself to just get on with it.

Your nervous system took notes.

And when the load became too much, it did what it was designed to do.

It tightened.

Many of the things you tried were not foolish. Some were sound. Some were sensible. But they were applied into a system that was already braced.

Fragments were treated. The whole was not.

Inflammation addressed.
Hormones adjusted.
Thoughts reframed.

But who checked whether you felt safe enough to receive any of it?

The hard truth?

You cannot bully a protective system into cooperation.

You cannot out-discipline a body that believes it is under threat.

And really, this is what I've found over and over again: when people stop fighting themselves, their physiology often changes before their protocol does.

Before trust returns—to medicine, to methods, or to your own body—safety must be re-established first.

Not positive thinking.

Not belief.

Not endurance.

Biological safety.

The quiet sense that nothing else is about to overwhelm you.

Without that, effort becomes friction.

With it, effort becomes integration.

So if you have been trying harder and getting worse, it does not mean you are failing.

It means your system has been protecting you.

And in the next chapter, we go to the place most approaches skip.

We start with safety.

Because once the body feels safe enough, it begins to listen again.

And when it listens, it can finally respond.

Chapter Three - When Treatments That Should Work Don't

You choose the treatment carefully.

It makes sense. It's well-designed. Well-reviewed. Properly explained. Finally, something structured. Something that sounds intelligent.

So you commit.

You follow it precisely. You take the doses on time. You attend the sessions. You change the food. You track the symptoms. You don't improvise. You don't cut corners.

For a few days—maybe a week—there's a lift.

The fog thins slightly. The pain eases. You feel just enough improvement to think, this might be it.

Then it fades.

By week three you feel worse than when you started. More tired. More wired. More fragile.

When you report this, you're encouraged to persist.

"It's part of the process."

"Stay the course."

So you do.

Until your body stops cooperating entirely.

And here's the hard part.

If you did everything right... why did it go wrong?

Repeated non-response dismantles your trust in cause and effect. You start to doubt the logic of effort. You begin to suspect the flaw is you.

Without an explanation, failure feels personal.

But biology doesn't reward compliance. It responds to conditions.

I once worked with a former nurse who had severe open leg ulcers. She understood wound care better than most professionals. The antibiotics were appropriate. The daily dressings were meticulous. Everything was correct.

And nothing healed.

Month after month the tissue remained open. No infection. No obvious error. Just no closure.

Then the conversation shifted. Surgery was raised. Wheelchair support discussed as a probable outcome if mobility declined further.

Same woman.

Same body.

And instead of feeling supported, she felt her world narrowing. Not expanding toward recovery —shrinking toward limitation.

She told me something that has stayed with me. The escalation felt like a threat, not a solution.

When the system remains unheard, intensifying intervention can feel like pressure rather than help.

What shifted for her wasn't a stronger protocol.

It was being listened to.

When we slowed everything down—when her experience was acknowledged instead of managed—her physiology began to settle. Not dramatically. Not overnight. But perceptibly.

Correct treatment does not guarantee biological receptivity.

That distinction changes everything.

Sometimes the issue isn't the treatment at all.

It's timing.

I worked with a man who wanted rapid functional improvement. Clear results. Measurable gains. When we began foundational regulation work—steady nervous system recalibration—he grew impatient. The changes were subtle. Systemic. Early-stage.

They didn't look impressive.

He left before the deeper work had time to stabilise.

Expectation shapes whether healing can be received. If you demand fruit before the roots have taken hold, you'll conclude nothing is growing.

And sometimes—this is uncomfortable—healing feels unsafe.

I remember a client whose breathing was chronically restricted. He manually controlled it throughout the day. It was his way of staying steady. As therapy reduced the tension driving the restriction, his breath began to regulate naturally.

Instead of relief, he felt panic.

If he wasn't controlling it, who was?

Control had become identity. When that control softened, he felt exposed. He withdrew rather than surrender the vigilance that had kept him feeling safe.

Your coping strategies are not random. They were intelligent adaptations. When therapy begins to dissolve them, the body can interpret that as danger.

So when treatments that should work don't, the

question is not, "What is wrong with me?"

It's this:

Was my system ready to receive this?

Was it safe enough?

Was the pace aligned with my biology—or with someone else's protocol?

When disappointment accumulates, hope becomes expensive. You start calculating emotional risk. You stop trying not because you've healed, but because you cannot afford another collapse.

I understand that.

When I worked inside highly structured medical environments, I saw how quickly non-response was framed as non-compliance. And I saw how damaging that narrative can be.

The body does not resist healing. It resists feeling unsafe.

Spring does not arrive because we insist on it. The soil warms. The light shifts. Conditions align.

Growth follows readiness.

What if your body isn't broken?

What if it's waiting for the right conditions?

Not stronger force.

Not more escalation.

But coherence.

Once that distinction becomes clear, you stop blaming yourself—and start asking better questions.

Signal Reception Theory™

At the beginning of this chapter, you met two people.

One was a former nurse with open leg ulcers that refused to close. As months passed, surgery was discussed. A wheelchair was introduced as a likely future support.

The other was a man who left early because progress did not arrive as quickly as he expected.

Different personalities.
Different clinical pictures.
Same underlying pattern.

Treatment that should have worked... didn't.

If everything is being done correctly, why am I not getting better?

The answer is rarely incompetence and rarely defiance.

It is often receptivity.

Receptivity Before Intervention

Let's return to the former nurse.

Her care was appropriate. Antibiotics were correct. Wound management was thorough. No obvious errors.

Still, the ulcers did not close.

Months later, the conversation shifted. Surgery. Escalation. Mobility aids. A narrowing horizon.

If correct treatment does not produce healing,

what do we assume?

Severity.
Failure.
Deterioration.

Sometimes the system is not deteriorating.

It is not receiving.

A body must be able to receive before it can respond.

When your nervous system is overloaded—chronic stress, disrupted sleep, years of disappointment, constant symptom monitoring—any new input is evaluated through a survival lens.

Is this safe?
Is this more demand?
Can I afford this?

If the answer is uncertain, the system tightens.

Overloaded systems interpret input as demand.

Even helpful input.

I have seen supplements meant to calm produce agitation. I have seen gentle protocols deepen fatigue. Not because they were inherently wrong, but because the system was already at capacity.

When I first understood this in my own life, it shifted everything. I stopped asking only, “Is this the right treatment?” and started asking, “Is my system able to receive this?”

That is a different conversation.

Guarded systems prioritise protection over repair.

Repair requires surplus.
Protection consumes it.

Timing Over Dosage

As her healing stalled, escalation was introduced.

Surgery was presented as responsible planning. Wheelchair support as pragmatic preparation.

Clinically defensible steps.

But from inside her body, it felt like contraction.

Escalation can feel like threat when the system remains unheard.

When a system feels threatened, it does not soften into repair.

It braces.

The usual response to stalled progress is intensity.

Increase the dose.
Add another intervention.
Accelerate the plan.

But readiness matters more than amount.

If input arrives before the system is ready, it triggers defence.

Biology moves in sequence.

Stabilisation first.
Repair second.
Optimisation last.

Reverse that order, and the body resists.

For the nurse, improvement did not begin with stronger intervention. It began when the pressure eased. When listening replaced urgency. When her system no longer felt pushed toward an inevitable outcome.

Safety returned first.

Then change.

That order matters.

Expectation Shapes Reception

Now consider the man who left early.

He wanted rapid improvement. Tangible results. A visible shift.

We began with foundational regulation work. Skin improved slightly. Temper softened. Small but meaningful gains.

Because the headline result had not yet arrived, he concluded it was ineffective.

He withdrew.

Early biological change is often subtle. It stabilises before it transforms.

But we are conditioned to look for dramatic relief.

If expectation outruns physiology, progress is abandoned too soon.

When receptivity is low, treatment stalls.
When timing is wrong, escalation backfires.
When expectation is impatient, healing is cut short.

None of that means the body is broken.

It means the system is protective.

Signal Clarity Over Intensity

When something doesn't work, we tend to add.

Another supplement.
Another therapy.
Another layer of effort.

But multiple inputs blur reception.

If your system is already managing energy like a

scarce currency—carefully calculating what you can afford before you crash—then every new intervention is another signal to interpret.

Interpretation costs energy.

And when energy is limited, clarity matters more than intensity.

I have seen people pause nearly everything—carefully, responsibly. Reduce to essentials. Simplify routines. Stabilise sleep and meals.

Symptoms soften.

Weeks later, something that previously "failed" works at half the dose.

Nothing changed about the intervention.

The signal environment changed.

Fewer signals often restore response.

Bringing It Back to You

If treatments that should have worked haven't worked for you, the conclusion is not automatically that you are resistant or beyond help.

It may mean:

Your system was overloaded.
The timing was misaligned.
The signal was too noisy.
The expectation was too urgent.

That is not a character flaw.

It is physiology.

Your body is not defying you. It is protecting you.

Protection softens when safety returns.

Perhaps nothing was "wrong" with the treatment.

Perhaps the signal simply could not be heard.

When Escalation Feels Logical — But Isn't

Let's be honest.

When something that should work doesn't, your

first instinct is not to slow down.

It's to try harder.

Increase the dose.
Add something "gentle."
Research longer.
Book another appointment.

You tell yourself you're being proactive.

Sometimes you're escalating because you're scared.

I've done it myself. When I've wanted relief quickly, I've layered interventions that made sense individually but overwhelmed the system collectively.

More effort does not equal more healing.

Sometimes it equals more noise.

So this week, we do something that feels almost rebellious.

We pause.

Not because you're giving up.
Not because nothing works.

But because your system may be too overloaded to receive.

Step One: Pause All New Interventions

For the next seven days, introduce nothing new.

No new supplements.
No new diets.
No new therapy bookings made late at night when hope spikes and fear whispers.

Just stop adding.

This sounds simple. It isn't.

The former nurse I mentioned earlier had months of correct antibiotics. Daily wound care. Every protocol followed precisely.

Nothing closed.

On paper, everything was right.

But her body was not responding.

As healing stalled, surgery was introduced. A wheelchair was discussed as a probable outcome. What began as treatment slowly felt like escalation. Her world started shrinking instead of expanding.

Correct treatment does not guarantee biological receptivity.

She didn't need more intervention first.

She needed her system to feel safe enough to receive.

When I sat with her—really listened—her physiology softened before the wound ever changed.

Healing is not just about correctness.

It is about cooperation.

You cannot cooperate with something when you feel pursued.

Step Two: Reduce to Essentials Only

Look at everything you're currently taking or doing.

Supplements.
Gut support.
Hormone support.
Sleep aids.
"Just in case" remedies.

Each one may be reasonable.

Together, they can be relentless.

This week, strip it back.

Keep prescribed medication exactly as directed.
Keep what is medically necessary.

But remove anything optional that creates agitation.

And be honest with yourself.

Does that supplement leave you wired?
Does that "gentle" therapy leave you shaky for days?
Is your sleep worse since you added it?

If yes, it comes out—for now.

You are not judging it.

You are clearing static.

Think of it like a pond after a storm. You can't see the bottom when everything is stirred.

Step Three: Remove Agitation

Agitation isn't always dramatic.

Sometimes it's subtle.

A racing mind.
Tight jaw.
Restless sleep.
Irritability you explain away.

You might have told yourself, "It's detox."
Or, "It gets worse before it gets better."

Sometimes that's true.

Sometimes that's rationalising overload.

Your nervous system reads intensity as threat, even when the intervention is well-intentioned.

This is where many people make the mistake.

They increase the dose to force a response.
They stack multiple "gentle" therapies.
They assume non-response means personal failure.

No.

Non-response is information.

It is not a verdict on you.

Step Four: Observe Without Correcting

This is the uncomfortable one.

When a symptom appears this week, don't immediately fix it.

Just watch.

How long does it last?
What came before it?
Does it rise and fall naturally?

You become curious instead of corrective.

The man who wanted rapid improvement came in focused, determined. He wanted measurable gains quickly.

We began with foundational regulation work. Nothing dramatic. Just stabilising the system.

He grew frustrated.

The early improvements were subtle. His sleep was slightly better. Reactivity reduced. But it wasn't the visible breakthrough he wanted.

He left too early.

Timing matters.

Expectation shapes perception.

If you're always scanning for outcome, you miss the early shifts.

Healing often starts quietly.

If you keep interrupting it, you never see it.

Step Five: Track Patterns, Not Outcomes

Don't ask, "Did I feel better today?"

Ask, "What happened around my symptoms?"

When do crashes happen?
After what kind of conversations?
After what kind of stimulation?
After pushing beyond your limit to look "functional"?

Use a simple notebook.

Morning energy score.
Sleep quality.
Major symptoms.
Stressors.

No analysis. No overthinking. Just notes.

Patterns tell the truth.

Outcomes fluctuate. Patterns reveal structure.

And here's something else you may notice.

You may feel safer when you are actively managing, fixing, controlling.

I once worked with a man who manually controlled his breathing almost constantly. Therapy gradually helped his body breathe more autonomously.

But when control reduced, panic increased.

Control was his safety.

Without it, he felt exposed.

Healing can feel unsafe when identity depends on control.

That's not weakness.

It's wiring.

And if you don't see it, you'll sabotage your own progress without meaning to.

Common Mistakes

Let me say these plainly.

Increasing the dose to force a reaction rarely works.
Stacking therapies because each one is "mild" still overloads the system.
Interpreting non-response as failure damages trust.

Sometimes nothing appears to be happening because your system is still bracing.

You cannot push a braced system into cooperation.

You can only reduce the pressure until it no longer feels threatened.

The 72-Hour Reset

If a week feels overwhelming, start with three days.

For 72 hours, pause optimisation.

No tweaking.
No adjusting.
No researching the next breakthrough.

Eat simply.
Sleep when tired.
Step outside once a day.
Limit stimulating conversations.

And just notice.

You are not trying to improve.

You are allowing recalibration.

When I've done this myself, the first thing I notice is fatigue. Real fatigue. The kind that surfaces when you finally stop performing resilience.

Then something else appears.

Quiet.

Subtle. Not dramatic.

But steady.

The body does not heal under interrogation.

It heals under conditions.

When treatments that should work don't work, it does not automatically mean you are broken.

It may mean you are overloaded.
It may mean you are unheard.
It may mean your system does not yet feel safe enough to receive.

That is not a life sentence.

It is a signal.

This week is not about fixing yourself.

It's about creating space for cooperation.

Less noise.
Less force.
More observation.

And in that space, something shifts.

Not loudly.

But honestly.

And sometimes, that is where everything begins to turn.

Closing Reflection

Let's say this plainly.

When treatments that should work don't work, it does something to you.

It's not just disappointment. It's erosion.

You begin to question your body. Your judgement. Your hope.

Non-response is often protective, not defective.

That can feel almost insulting when you are exhausted. You followed instructions. You endured side effects. You kept going when you wanted to stop.

And still—nothing.

You have been taught that correct input should produce correct output. That is how research is designed. Control the variables. Apply the intervention. Measure the change.

But you are not a controlled trial.

You are a living system.

Living systems respond to safety, not pressure.

Treatment correctness does not ensure biological receptivity.

You can apply the right intervention to a system that is still braced, and it will not integrate. Not because it cannot. But because it does not yet feel safe enough to.

Have you noticed how your body reacts when a new "next step" is suggested? Even when it sounds reasonable? A subtle tightening. A quiet internal recoil.

Escalation can look logical. In the body, it can register as threat.

When a system feels pushed, it protects.

Reception determines outcome.

Reception is shaped by timing.

You may have experienced small improvements—slightly deeper sleep, a calmer morning, less volatility in your symptoms. But because those changes were not dramatic, you may have dismissed them.

Healing often begins below the level of spectacle.

It is like tuning an old radio. At first there is static. You turn the dial slightly. Still static. You adjust again. A faint signal flickers through, then disappears.

It would be easy to say nothing is happening.

But something is.

You are moving toward coherence.

If you twist the dial too aggressively because you cannot yet hear the music, you overshoot the frequency entirely.

Timing matters more than effort.

You cannot rush alignment.

And then there is control.

If you have lived with unpredictable symptoms, you have likely become highly vigilant. You monitor. You plan. You calculate. That vigilance has kept you functional.

But here is the harder reality.

Healing can feel unsafe when identity is organised around control.

Remember the man I mentioned earlier whose breathing felt permanently restricted. He manually regulated every breath to prevent panic. It was exhausting, but it gave him a sense of control. As therapy gently reduced the need for that constant management, something unexpected happened.

His panic increased.

Not because he was deteriorating.

But because control was loosening.

The mechanism that had protected him for years was being softened. And that felt dangerous.

When coping strategies become identity, healing can feel like threat.

If you have built your life around managing symptoms—tracking food, rationing energy, anticipating crashes—who are you without that vigilance?

That question alone can activate fear.

When I have reduced my own over-control in certain areas of life, I have felt that flicker of anxiety. The space feels too open at first. Too unstructured. The body prefers the familiar, even when the familiar is exhausting.

Subtraction restores capacity.

But subtraction often feels like loss before it feels like relief.

Less monitoring. Less bracing. Less constant adjusting.

It feels exposed.

So if treatments have not worked for you, pause before deciding your body is defective.

Ask a different question.

Did your system feel ready?
Did it feel resourced?
Did it feel safe enough to shift?

Because here is what most approaches overlook.

Readiness is not psychological.
It is biological.

You cannot think yourself into receptivity.
You cannot discipline yourself into integration.
You cannot optimise your way out of protection.

If the nervous system detects threat, even subtle threat, it will prioritise defence over repair every time.

That is not resistance.

That is intelligence.

The body does not respond to force.

It responds to conditions.

And if conditions have not been aligned, then escalating treatment will continue to feel like pressure.

What you have been calling "non-response" may simply be protection waiting for stability.

This is where most healing models stop.

They focus on the intervention.

They rarely stabilise the terrain.

In the next chapter, we move underneath the protocol.

We examine the system that decides whether any treatment is received at all.

Because before receptivity comes regulation.

Before regulation comes safety.

And safety is not a mindset.

It is a physiological state.

When that state shifts, everything else becomes possible.

Chapter Four - When Talking Can Make the Body Worse

You go to the session because you genuinely want to get better.

You are not avoiding your life.
You are not in denial.
You are trying.

You sit down. You talk. You connect the dots. You understand yourself more clearly than you ever have before.

And then you go home.

By evening your body feels worse.

The fatigue is thicker. The pain sharper. Your sleep breaks into small, brittle pieces. You lie there wondering, *How can insight make me feel this ill?*

You are told this is normal. "It's part of healing." "It has to get worse before it gets better."

But the truth is... your body does not experience it as progress. It experiences it as load.

A pattern becomes clear when you look closely: emotional insight and physical capacity are not the same thing. You can understand more than your nervous system can safely carry.

And when the volume of emotion exceeds the body's ability to regulate it, symptoms rise.

Not because you are weak.
Not because you are resistant.
Because your system is trying to stabilise.

I remember a woman who described leaving counselling sessions with what she called "a bag of sorrows." During the hour she felt lighter. Seen. Heard. Validated.

But each session unearthed more material. More memories. More grief. More anger.

Insight accumulated. Stability did not.

Within a short time she was exhausted. Her symptoms flared. Her sleep deteriorated. She began to dread the sessions that were meant to help her.

Processing without containment increases

burden.

That is uncomfortable to admit. But it matters.

When your system is already stretched by chronic fatigue or pain, emotional excavation can feel like another demand. Another task. Another stressor.

Have you ever noticed yourself calculating what you can afford to talk about?

I have. When I was younger in my own reflective work, I could feel when I had opened too much. There is a tipping point. A subtle internal "enough." When I ignored it, I paid for it physically.

The woman with the "bag of sorrows" learned something important. Some sessions she chose not to speak about everything. She allowed silence.

Silence.

Not avoidance. Not denial. Regulation.

She left steadier. She slept better. Her body responded to the restraint.

The truth is... sometimes silence is intelligence.

You may have done this yourself. Held something back. Changed the subject. Skimmed the surface.

And then wondered if that meant you were failing at therapy.

It may have meant you were protecting your nervous system.

That distinction changes everything.

Then there was the man who phoned about his digestion. He spoke at length, primarily wanting his interpretation confirmed. Instead of analysing symptoms in detail, I gently reflected something simple: digestion is not only about food. It is about how we process experience.

There was a pause.

He reconsidered the story he was telling himself. He never became a client. He did not need to. Recognition alone shifted something.

No excavation. No reliving. No emotional flood.

Just orientation.

Really, this is what I've found... the body does not always need more exposure. Sometimes it needs coherence. Sometimes it needs safety first.

When emotional work worsens your physical symptoms, two things often happen.

You blame yourself.

Or you walk away from support altogether.

You think, *I must be blocked.*
Or you think, *Nothing helps me.*

Both reactions are understandable.

But the truth is... the problem may not be your willingness. It may be pacing.

We have been taught that talking is always good. That expression is inherently healing.

Often, it is.

But when the nervous system is already unsettled, talking can amplify signal rather than settle it. The body does not always distinguish between remembering and reliving unless it feels safe enough to do so.

And safety is not a mindset. It is a physiological state.

So if you have ever left a session feeling worse—more inflamed, more exhausted, more fragile—please hear this clearly:

You are not broken.
You are not doing it wrong.

Your system may simply need containment before excavation.

Stability before story.
Regulation before revelation.

The body is not opposed to truth.

It is opposed to overload.

When you understand that, something softens. You stop associating awareness with harm. You stop shaming yourself for needing a slower pace.

And that, quietly, is where trust begins to return.

The Somatic Safety Principle™

Earlier in this chapter, you met the woman who described therapy as carrying a bag of sorrows.

And you met the man with digestive pain who was, perhaps, struggling to "stomach" his own narrative.

Those stories were not random.

They were not illustrations.

They were clues.

Now we slow down and look at what they were really showing us.

Because the truth is, talking can make the body worse.

Not always.

But often enough — especially when the

nervous system is already sensitised.

You have probably been told the opposite.
Speak it and you release it.
Understand it and you dissolve it.

And yet, your symptoms did not improve.

You talked.
You reflected.
You understood.

But your fatigue stayed.
Your flares continued.
Your body tightened the next day.

Why?

your body does not heal because it understands.

It heals when it feels safe.

the nervous system follows biology, not intention.

You can want insight.
You can crave resolution.
You can be courageous in conversation.

But if your system still detects threat, reflection becomes activation.

And activation, in a sensitised body, becomes symptoms.

This is the foundation of the Somatic Safety Principle™.

Safety before insight.
Containment over catharsis.
Non-talking first.

Let's return to the woman with the bag.

Step 1: Safety Before Insight

In the opening, you saw how her therapy sessions left her heavier.

Now look at it physiologically.

Each time she unpacked grief, her nervous system activated. Not because she was weak. But because memory is not abstract. The body replays elements of the original state.

Heart rate shifts.

Muscle tone increases.
Stress chemistry pulses.

In a robust system, this activation resolves.

In a sensitised system — like hers, like yours may be — it lingers.

Lingering activation becomes flare.

The bag of sorrows was not metaphorical. It was physiological load.

Insight was increasing.

Capacity was not.

Really, this is what I've found again and again — the nervous system does not prioritise meaning. It prioritises survival. If it senses overwhelm, it responds defensively.

Safety must precede insight.

Not because insight is wrong.

But because biology sets the order.

Step 2: Containment Over Catharsis

In the opening, you also saw her make a subtle shift.

She chose silence.

Not avoidance.

Not resistance.

But regulation.

What you may not have seen yet is why that mattered so much.

She began to notice that on weeks when she pushed through — when she excavated more — her migraines intensified.

So she experimented.

Mid-session, when she felt that internal escalation — tight chest, rising intensity, that familiar edge — she stopped.

She limited disclosure.

She protected her bandwidth.

And something changed.

Her flares reduced.
Her sleep steadied.
The bag stopped growing so quickly.

First, you saw the weight accumulating.

Then you saw her instinctively choose containment.

That is not regression.

That is intelligence.

catharsis without capacity destabilises.

Your nervous system measures intensity, not bravery. If emotional disclosure exceeds tolerance, the body defends.

Containment preserves capacity.

Really, this is what I've found — dramatic release feels productive. But steadiness builds resilience.

And when you live with chronic illness, resilience is the currency that matters.

Step 3: Non-Talking First

Now consider the man you met earlier — the one with digestive complaints.

On the surface, he wanted treatment.

But what became clear was that he was holding tightly to his narrative. He wanted confirmation.

Instead of offering intervention, I reflected something simple: digestion is about breaking down and assimilating. What, in your life, are you struggling to stomach?

There was a pause.

No catharsis.

No deep excavation.

Just recognition.

He did not need more processing.

He needed perspective — delivered without activation.

And that is the thread linking his story with hers.

When the nervous system is overloaded, more material increases strain.

When the nervous system is steady, even small insight can integrate cleanly.

Regulation precedes narrative.

Always.

The woman eventually paused trauma processing entirely for a while. She stabilised sleep. Reduced stimulation. Focused on regulation before reflection.

Her symptoms softened.

Only later did she reintroduce limited insight work — this time within a steadier baseline.

Bodies stabilise before minds integrate.

This is not ideology.

It is biology.

the nervous system follows biology, not intention.

Why This Matters For You

If you are already living near threshold — disrupted sleep, chronic inflammation, unpredictable flares — your margin for activation is narrow.

Talking about trauma activates neural networks associated with the original event. In a resilient system, that resolves.

In a sensitised one, it lingers.

Lingering activation becomes flare.

This is why you may leave therapy feeling heard... yet wake exhausted.

It is not weakness.

It is order.

The same stories you encountered at the beginning of this chapter were not cautionary tales.

They were demonstrations of sequence.

The bag grew when safety was missing.

Silence stabilised when containment was introduced.

Recognition shifted perspective when activation was low.

Insight is not the enemy.

Poor sequencing is.

Safety before insight.
Containment over catharsis.
Non-talking first.

Really, this is what I've found consistently — when safety increases, symptoms often soften. When containment strengthens, resilience grows. When regulation leads, insight integrates instead of inflames.

You are not failing at therapy.

Your body is asking for the right order.

And when you honour that order, healing stops feeling like effort.

It begins to feel like stability.

Implementation is not dramatic.

It is not a breakthrough conversation.
It is not finally saying the thing you have never said.

It is quieter than that.

It starts with this question:

What is actually helping your body — consistently?

Not what sounds clever.
Not what works once.
Not what makes sense on paper.

What leaves you steadier tomorrow?

Really, this is what I've found... the body keeps score of stability, not insight.

You have probably spent years trying to solve yourself. Analysing. Interpreting. Explaining. I understand that instinct. When I first stepped out of formal research environments and into clinical practice, I was trained to look for mechanisms, causes, correlations. Find the driver. Fix it.

But the truth is... physiology does not reorganise because you understand it. It reorganises because it feels safe enough to shift.

So begin here.

Notice what works.

Maybe it is eating at the same time every day.
Maybe it is stopping work before you feel exhausted rather than after.
Maybe it is declining a conversation that you know will cost you three days.

These are not small things.

They are regulatory anchors.

And your nervous system is desperate for anchors.

Now, let me connect something important.

You may remember the woman I described earlier — the one who left counselling sessions temporarily soothed but physiologically heavier. She was thoughtful. Insightful. Committed to the process. She wanted to heal properly.

Every week she unpacked more. Childhood memories. Relationship dynamics. Hidden resentments.

And every week she left carrying what she later described as "a bag of sorrows."

The conversations were not wrong. The therapist was not wrong.

But her capacity to hold what was uncovered had not expanded.

Processing increased. Containment did not.

The truth is... when emotional excavation outpaces physiological stability, symptoms often intensify.

Over time, she noticed something. On weeks

when she said less, she felt better afterwards. Not emotionally triumphant. But physically steadier.

So she experimented.

She chose silence.

Not as avoidance. Not as denial. But as regulation.

She spoke only what she could carry home without tipping her system into overload.

Really, this is what I've found... silence can sometimes be the most intelligent intervention.

You are allowed to pace your own disclosure.
You are allowed to limit what you process in one sitting.
You are allowed to protect your nervous system.

Stop chasing fixes.

Chasing keeps you in a forward-leaning posture — subtly braced, subtly urgent.

You can feel it, can't you? That internal push. The sense that if you just find the right supplement, the right therapist, the right protocol, everything will finally unlock.

I have seen that urgency many times. I have felt it myself in other areas of life. When I have wanted certainty, I have sometimes rushed toward answers just to quiet the discomfort of not knowing.

But the truth is... urgency and safety rarely coexist.

Before you begin something new, pause.

Ask: Am I building stability, or am I trying to outrun uncertainty?

There is a difference.

Honour small gains.

You may dismiss them. Please don't.

One night of deeper sleep.
One afternoon without a crash.
One conversation that didn't spike your heart rate.

These are not trivial. They are data.

When I worked in clinical research, change was never judged by one dramatic moment. It was judged by pattern. Trend. Direction.

Your body works the same way.

Keep it simple. At the end of each day, write down one thing your body did right.

Digestion that felt smoother.
Muscles that relaxed more quickly.
A wave of emotion that passed without flooding you.

This is not positive thinking. It is pattern recognition.

And really, this is what I've found... when you start noticing cooperation instead of failure, your nervous system softens.

Now let me bring in the man who called about his digestive problems.

He had symptoms, yes. But what he wanted most was validation of his story — why it was happening, what it meant, how it proved something about his past.

As he spoke, I gently reflected something simple: digestion is the body's ability to break down, assimilate, and discard. What, I asked him, was he struggling to "digest" in his life?

There was a pause.

You could hear the recognition land.

He did not need a treatment plan in that moment. He needed awareness.

He never became a client. But he left reconsidering his internal dialogue.

Recognition alone shifted something.

The same principle runs through all of these people — and perhaps through you.

The woman who over-processed and chose silence to stabilise.
The man who realised he was struggling to digest experience, not just food.

The thread is capacity.

Insight without capacity overwhelms.

Expression without containment destabilises.
Narrative without regulation exhausts.

Reduce contingency planning.

I know why you do it.

You calculate energy before committing. You imagine the crash before it happens. You prepare exit strategies.

It makes sense. When I have lived through periods of depletion, I have done the same. Planning feels protective.

But constant anticipation keeps your system rehearsing threat.

Try this gently.

Choose one small activity this week without building three backup plans. Give yourself permission to leave early — but don't pre-live the collapse.

See what actually happens.

Allow cautious hope.

Not blind optimism. Not magical thinking.

Measured hope.

If you notice that pacing helps... that silence sometimes protects you... that small gains accumulate...

Then hope is not delusion.

It is evidence-based.

You may still make mistakes.

You may demand certainty before relaxing.
You may rush progress the moment you feel better.
You may compare yourself to who you were ten years ago and feel grief.

That grief is real.

But the truth is... comparison to your past capacity keeps you anchored in loss, not direction.

Ask a different question.

Am I slightly more regulated than last month?

Not perfect. Not cured.

Just steadier.

Before you close this chapter tonight, pause.

Notice one thing your body did right today.

Just one.

Because really, this is what I've found… when you shift from trying to fix yourself to learning how to stabilise yourself, something profound begins to happen.

Your body stops defending.

And starts reorganising.

There is something we are rarely told.

Insight is not neutral.

You can understand your history in exquisite detail. You can name your triggers. You can map your relationships and explain your patterns with intelligence and grace.

And still feel worse.

Over time, a pattern became impossible to ignore... awareness does not automatically create regulation. sometimes it does the opposite. Sometimes it activates a body that was already stretched thin.

Have you ever left a conversation feeling emotionally “clear” but physically unsettled? Tired. Wired. Slightly unwell. As though something had been opened but not integrated.

That is not weakness. It is physiology.

Safety always precedes processing. Not as a philosophy. As biology.

When I began to observe this more closely in my own work, it changed how I listened. I would see people gaining insight week after week, yet their sleep declined. Their digestion tightened. Their pain intensified. And I had to ask myself a harder question.

Was more talking actually helping?

Here’s what became clear... if your nervous

system does not feel safe, processing becomes another stressor. It is like renovating a house in the middle of a storm. The effort itself destabilises the structure.

The body measures safety first. Not insight. Not catharsis. Not how bravely you told the story.

If your system is already overwhelmed, digging deeper can increase the load.

And this is the part that can feel uncomfortable: sometimes silence is not avoidance. It is intelligence.

When I have felt emotionally overloaded myself, I have chosen to say less. Not because I was in denial. Not because I lacked courage. But because I knew my capacity was limited that day. When I honoured that limit, my system stabilised more quickly.

Have you ever sensed that opening one more door would tip you into collapse?

That instinct is not pathology. It is preservation.

We have been culturally conditioned to believe

that more disclosure equals more healing. That bravery looks like endless excavation. But the physiology tells us something simpler. Timing matters more than intensity.

Less talking can restore regulation.

Why? Because it reduces stimulation. It lowers cognitive demand. It allows your system to experience an hour without defending, remembering, explaining, or justifying.

And sometimes that is enough.

Bodies heal without stories.

This does not mean stories are irrelevant. It means the body does not require constant narration to reorganise itself. Your heart beats without explanation. Your skin repairs without discussion. Your gut recalibrates without a detailed autobiography.

What consistently reveals itself is this... when safety returns, clarity follows.

Not forced clarity. Not analytical clarity. A quieter one.

You think more slowly. You feel less urgency. Decisions simplify. You stop chasing understanding because your system is no longer bracing.

The reality is, many chronically unwell people are not failing at therapy. They are exceeding their capacity.

Capacity can be rebuilt.

But it is rebuilt through regulation, not repetition.

You are not broken because talking exhausted you. You are not resistant because your body tightened when sessions went deeper. You may simply have needed stabilisation before exploration.

Once safety returns, clarity becomes possible again.

Not because you tried harder. Not because you told the story better.

But because your body finally felt secure enough to soften.

And softness, in a system that has been on guard for years, is not weakness.

It is the beginning of coherence.

Chapter Five - Clearing the Fog - Why Your Brain Is Not Broken

It often begins quietly.

Standing in the kitchen, staring at food, and not knowing what to choose.
Not because there are no options. But because the decision feels strangely heavy.

Emails get read more than once. Then again.
Rooms are entered, and the reason for being there slips away.
A sentence starts... and the right word does not arrive.

There is a pause. A flicker of unease.

And then the question surfaces.

What if something is wrong?
What if this is decline?

Tests come back normal. Blood work steady. Nothing alarming.

And yet, something feels different.

The truth is, this kind of mental fog unsettles people in a very particular way. It is not just about inconvenience. It touches identity. It raises a quiet fear that something essential is slipping.

Who am I if I cannot think clearly?

Here is something I've come to understand over years of clinical observation... most people who feel this way are not experiencing a failing brain. They are experiencing a system under strain.

The brain does not operate in isolation. It depends on energy, oxygen, and a sense of safety. When the body is stretched, the brain adapts.

Clear thinking takes effort.
Quick decisions take effort.
Finding the right words takes effort.

And when the system senses pressure — whether physical or emotional — it reduces what is not immediately necessary.

Not dramatically. Subtly.

I worked with a senior executive who described this with striking clarity. Highly capable, respected, used to holding complex information with ease. And then, during a board meeting, she lost her words.

Not a small stumble. A complete blank.

She could see what she wanted to say, but could not access it.

Her fear was immediate. Not just embarrassment — but something deeper. A sense that her authority was slipping.

Medical tests showed nothing concerning. No neurological issue. But the problem continued, particularly in high-stakes situations.

Over time, a pattern emerged.

What became clear to me was this... brain fog is often linked to perceived pressure, not damage.

Her thinking faltered most in environments where she felt scrutinised or not fully heard. Where she had to brace, even slightly.

And bracing has a cost.

The part of the brain responsible for decisions, language, and clarity works best when the body feels safe. If the system is on alert, that clarity is quietly reduced.

Not because something is broken.

Because something is protecting.

She noticed another shift. In rooms where she felt respected, where there was steadiness, her clarity returned. No special techniques. No cognitive training.

Just a change in environment.

This is something I've seen repeatedly... mental clarity often follows a sense of safety.

Earlier in my career, I saw similar patterns in clinical settings. Capable professionals would lose fluency under pressure, then regain it as soon as the atmosphere softened. Their knowledge had not disappeared. It had simply become harder to access.

Context matters more than most people realise.

There may be a recognition here. Perhaps the fog worsens in appointments where there is a need to explain or defend. Perhaps it deepens in conversations where there is a subtle sense of not being believed.

And this is where a harder truth sits.

When someone feels dismissed, the body responds. Not emotionally alone, but physically. Thinking narrows. Words become harder to find.

The system withdraws.

Over time, this begins to change behaviour.

Decisions are delayed.
Choices are second-guessed.
Complexity is avoided.

Life becomes smaller. Not all at once, but gradually.

This is how cognitive fatigue erodes confidence. And with that, independence begins to slip.

But there is another way to look at this.

From what I have consistently observed... this fog is rarely a sign of failure. It is more often a sign of overload.

Imagine a tree in winter. From the outside, it appears still, even lifeless. But internally, it is conserving. Protecting. Waiting.

Nothing is broken.

The body does something similar.

When demands have been high for too long, when energy has been stretched, when the system has not felt fully safe, the brain begins to conserve. It slows what is not essential in the moment.

Not permanently. Just for now.

So the question shifts.

What if this is not decline...
but protection?

Forcing clarity rarely works. Pushing harder often deepens the fog.

But when the conditions change — when there

is steadiness, when there is enough energy, when the system no longer needs to brace — something else begins to happen.

Clarity returns.

Not because it was rebuilt.
Because it was never gone.

It was waiting for the right conditions.

The Cognitive Load Reset™

Let's say this plainly.

Brain fog is frightening.

Not because you misplace your keys.
But because you misplace your confidence.

You used to think quickly. Speak clearly. Hold complexity without strain. And now?

You lose words mid-sentence.
You reread messages twice.
You walk into a room and pause.

And a quiet thought surfaces:

Is this decline?
Is something wrong with my brain?

The truth is... brain fog is far more often overload than damage.

What I've come to understand over time is this... when the system is carrying too much, clarity is the first thing to dim.

Not because you are broken.
Because your brain is prioritising survival.

And once you see that, the story begins to change.

Step 1 — Reduce Signal Traffic

Have you ever tried to speak in a crowded room?

Music in the background. Multiple conversations. Movement everywhere. Your hearing works. Your language works. But you strain. You guess. You nod when you're not entirely sure what was said.

That isn't deafness.

That's traffic.

Brain fog works the same way.

When you live with ongoing symptoms, your brain processes more than anyone sees.

Pain signals.
Inflammation.
Sleep disruption.
Hormonal shifts.
Gut instability.
Medication effects.
Energy calculations.

And then life on top of that.

Work. Family. Deadlines. Social expectations. The effort of appearing capable. The quiet management of your own fear.

And beneath it all? Vigilance.

Monitoring your body.
Predicting crashes.
Preparing explanations.
Anticipating disbelief.

That's not weakness.
That's load.

If I'm being completely honest... most people who fear cognitive decline are actually experiencing cognitive congestion.

When I began observing this pattern, I saw it across genders, roles, and ages. Intelligent, capable men and women convinced they were deteriorating. But when I looked closely, I didn't see failing brains. I saw overwhelmed systems.

And overwhelmed systems slow down.

Why this works:
Your brain has limited processing bandwidth. Every incoming signal competes for attention. When there are too many, your system prioritises threat detection and stability over nuanced thinking. Switching between inputs burns energy. Excess switching creates that heavy, sticky sensation you call fog.

Reduce input.
Reduce switching.
Free capacity.

Clarity often returns not because you trained your brain, but because you stopped crowding it.

This brings us back to the executive from the opening of this chapter — the leader who suddenly lost their words in a high-stakes meeting.

Let's connect this properly.

In that boardroom moment, language faltered. Sentences stalled. Thoughts felt thick. It wasn't lack of intelligence. It was load.

The brain was scanning.

Scanning tone.
Scanning faces.
Scanning status.
Scanning for threat.

Because underneath the performance pressure was something more primal: exposure.

And exposure activates protection.

Step 2 — Eliminate Decision Drain

Here is a harder truth.

Chronic illness turns you into a constant decision-maker.

What to eat.
When to rest.
Whether you can manage today.
Whether to cancel.
Whether to push through.
Whether you are imagining symptoms.
Whether you can trust your own perception.

Most of these decisions are small.
None of them are neutral.

When the body feels unpredictable, every choice carries risk.

Will this make me worse?

That question alone consumes energy.

When I went through a season of sustained stress myself, I remember standing in my kitchen paralysed by simple decisions. Tea or coffee. Email now or later. It wasn't the complexity of the choice. It was the accumulation.

The truth is... deliberation is expensive.

Every time you weigh options, you use working memory and metabolic energy. When your system is already strained, constant micro-decisions drain the very cognitive resources you are trying to protect.

One thing I've seen again and again... fog deepens when life requires endless negotiation.

Why this works:
Automation conserves energy. When routines pre-decide for you, the brain does less comparative processing. Fewer internal debates mean fewer background calculations. That frees working memory for actual thinking.

This is not about rigidity.
It's about conservation.

Now let's connect this to the second part of the executive's story.

After the boardroom incident, something became clear. The fog wasn't random. It intensified in specific relational contexts — especially when this person felt unheard or subtly undermined.

When they felt dismissed.

When their reality was questioned.
When they had to defend their competence.

In those moments, cognition dimmed again.

Not emotionally.
Neurologically.

The truth is... not being believed is physiologically destabilising.

When you feel unsafe in a relational environment, your nervous system reallocates resources toward protection. Nuanced thinking, word retrieval, and fluid reasoning drop in priority. Scanning and bracing rise.

That shift can happen in seconds.

As relational safety improved — as they were genuinely listened to and taken seriously — clarity returned. Not gradually through cognitive training. Not through memory exercises.

Through safety.

If there's one pattern I trust in clinical work, it's this... mental clarity follows psychological safety more reliably than it follows intellectual effort.

Step 3 — Restore Predictability

If overload is the storm, predictability is the harbour.

Not control.
Not perfection.
Just rhythm.

When your body behaves unpredictably, your brain remains on watch. Watchfulness is not the same as clarity. It is vigilance.

Have you noticed how fog worsens when your days are chaotic?

Irregular meals.
Erratic sleep.
Last-minute changes.
Emotional unpredictability.

Your system never stands down.

The truth is... unpredictability keeps cognition in survival mode.

Why this works:

Predictable rhythms reduce perceived threat. When the nervous system expects what comes next, it stops scanning constantly. Reduced scanning frees processing capacity. Working memory stabilises. Word retrieval improves. Focus lengthens.

Something as simple as eating at regular times can sharpen thinking. Not because food is a miracle solution, but because physiological stability reduces background alarms.

When I stabilised my own daily rhythms during an intense period of work, I noticed something subtle. My thinking felt less interrupted. Not dramatically faster — just smoother. More coherent.

That's often how clarity returns. Quietly. Gradually. Reliably.

For the executive, once daily routines were simplified and relational safety strengthened, the fog reduced significantly. Authority returned — not through force, but through coherence.

Real-World Application — Fog Lifts Without Brain Training

Now imagine this in your life.

You reduce signal traffic.
Fewer unnecessary inputs.
Less constant information consumption.
Less self-monitoring that spirals.

You eliminate decision drain.
Defaults for meals.
Defaults for mornings.
Simplified choices where possible.

You restore predictability.
Regular sleep windows.
Regular nourishment.
Consistent rhythms.

Not to shrink your life.
To stabilise it.

And then something begins to shift.

You finish a sentence without searching.
You read a page and absorb it.
You enter a room and remember why.

Small moments.
But powerful.

The truth is... clarity often returns when load reduces.

Not because you fought harder.
But because you carried less.

This book is for anyone who has quietly feared they are slipping away — whether you are leading a company, managing a household, building a career, caring for others, or simply trying to remain yourself.

Brain fog does not discriminate by gender.
But overload is universal.

And overload has levers.

Time and again, this is what becomes clear... when you reduce traffic, decision drain, and unpredictability, the brain often remembers how to think clearly.

Not because it was repaired.
Because it was relieved.

Let's be honest.

When your brain feels unreliable, it is frightening.

You lose a word mid-sentence. You walk into a room and forget why. You reread the same paragraph three times. And somewhere in the back of your mind a harder thought appears:

What if this is decline?

The truth is... that fear alone can thicken the fog.

From years of observing this pattern, one thing becomes clear. Brain fog is rarely a sign that your mind is broken. It is usually a sign that your system feels under pressure.

And pressure changes priorities.

When the body senses threat—whether from blood sugar swings, emotional tension, overwork, or feeling dismissed—it diverts energy away from nuanced thinking. Articulation drops down the list. Memory softens. Precision wavers.

Not because you are failing.

Because your biology is protecting you.

So instead of training your brain harder, we reduce the load it is carrying.

Let me show you what that looks like in real life.

1. Standardise Your Meals

This may sound almost too simple.

But your brain is an energy-intensive organ. It runs on stability.

When I began paying attention to my own cognitive dips, I noticed something uncomfortable. On days I skipped meals or ate erratically, my thinking suffered. Not dramatically. Just enough to feel less sharp. Less steady.

The truth is... unstable fuel creates unstable clarity.

So simplify.

Choose two or three breakfasts you rotate. Eat at roughly the same times each day. Build lunches that are predictable and balanced rather than exciting and experimental.

You are not dieting.

You are reducing uncertainty.

When your body trusts that nourishment is coming, it relaxes. And when it relaxes, your brain can afford to think again.

Small rhythm. Big impact.

2. Reduce Daily Decisions

Decision fatigue is real. And when you are already managing symptoms, it accumulates fast.

How many micro-choices do you make before midday? What to wear. What to eat. Which email to answer first. Whether to rest or push through.

Each one costs something.

What becomes evident over time is this... clarity often returns when demand drops.

You may remember the executive I introduced earlier in this chapter, who lost her words mid-boardroom. The moment wasn't subtle. It was sharp. Public. Disorienting.

This was not a woman lacking intelligence. She had built her reputation on clarity. On precision. On being able to hold complexity without strain.

And yet, there she was. Pausing. Searching. Blank.

She told me later the silence felt louder than any mistake.

At first, she feared neurological decline. That something irreversible had begun. But as we explored further—just as we began to unpack in Chapter 5—another pattern revealed itself.

Her environment had changed. Leadership instability. Public scrutiny. Decisions being questioned in real time.

She no longer felt secure in the room.

And here is the part most people miss.

Her fog intensified when she felt unheard. When her input was dismissed. When she sensed doubt from others.

The truth is... not being believed shuts cognition down.

Her brain wasn't failing. It was reallocating.

Once relational safety improved—clearer roles, fewer unnecessary meetings, direct conversations—her clarity returned. No cognitive retraining. No apps.

Just less perceived threat.

This is the thread that runs through both her story and yours.

So ask yourself:

Where are you making unnecessary decisions? Where can you create defaults?

Wear similar outfits during the week. Batch your food planning. Decide once instead of ten times.

One less decision is one more ounce of clarity.

3. Limit Information Intake

This one is hard.

When you feel unwell, you search. You research. You join forums. You compare protocols. It feels proactive.

But be honest.

How often does it leave you calmer?

The truth is... too much information can feel like danger.

Your nervous system does not distinguish between a physical threat and relentless, contradictory input. Both increase vigilance.

I have done this myself. When I've dived too deeply into research late at night, I can feel the shift. My body tightens. My thoughts race. Clarity drops.

Over time, a consistent pattern emerges... the more input you carry, the less space your mind has to organise itself.

So create boundaries.

Give yourself a defined window for health research. Then close it. Step away from symptom discussions that leave you feeling dismissed or frightened.

Curate your inputs like you curate your food.

Because your brain reflects what it is swimming in.

4. Single-Task

Multitasking sounds efficient.

It isn't.

It is constant switching. And switching drains.

If you are writing, just write. If you are eating, just eat. Close tabs. Silence notifications. Set a short timer and commit to one task only.

When I began doing this intentionally, I noticed something subtle but powerful. My thoughts felt smoother. Less fragmented. I wasn't working harder. I was working with less interference.

Coherence returns confidence.

Confidence reduces threat.

And reduced threat restores cognition.

It really is that circular.

5. Build Predictable Routines

Your nervous system loves rhythm.

Wake at a similar time. Anchor your mornings. Close your evenings in the same way—dim lights, familiar music, a repeated sequence.

Predictability is not boring. It is stabilising.

Think of nature. The tide does not negotiate its timing each day. Seasons do not improvise randomly. Pattern conserves energy.

When your days become less chaotic, your brain stops scanning so intensely.

And scanning is what creates fog.

Common Mistakes

When clarity dips, it is tempting to fix it aggressively.

Brain-training apps.
More supplements.
Forcing longer focus sessions.

The truth is... if your system feels unsafe, adding more cognitive demand can make things worse.

Information overload is another trap. Ten new strategies at once fragment attention further.

And pushing through exhaustion? That often ends in a crash.

Instead of adding, try subtracting.

What can you remove today?

A Simple Experiment

Choose one thing to stop deciding.

Just one.

It might be breakfast. It might be your work outfit. It might be saying no to one unnecessary commitment.

Notice what happens.

Time and again, I've seen this... clarity often returns quietly. Not because something dramatic changed. But because pressure eased.

Your brain is not broken.

It has been managing more than you realised.

When you are believed, when fuel is steady, when demands soften, when rhythm returns—the fog thins.

Not all at once.

But enough for you to recognise yourself again.

And that is where real confidence begins.

Let's come back to something steady.

Your brain is not broken.

It is overwhelmed. It is cautious. It is doing exactly what a well-designed nervous system does when life feels unpredictable.

The truth is, fog is not failure. It is protection.

I have seen this pattern more times than I can count. What has become clear over time is this... when the body feels under pressure, the brain turns down the volume on everything that is not essential. Sophisticated language. Sharp recall. Fast thinking. These are not survival priorities.

You remember the executive I told you about. The CEO who lost her words mid-meeting.

She had always been articulate. Quick. Commanding. Then one morning, in front of her board, her vocabulary thinned. She could see the information in her mind, but she could not retrieve it cleanly. Her authority felt as though it were slipping through her fingers.

What frightened her was not dementia. It was humiliation.

As we explored further, something else emerged. It was not just workload. It was not just hormones. Her cognitive dips intensified when she felt doubted. Interrupted. Quietly undermined.

It was the same woman. The same boardroom. The same brain.

But two different environments inside her body.

When she felt scrutinised, her words scattered. When she felt respected and supported, her clarity returned—without brain games, without memory drills, without forcing anything.

That is not coincidence.

Not being believed shuts cognition down. Feeling safe opens it back up.

The truth is, your brain does not perform well under threat. Even subtle threat. Especially subtle threat.

Have you noticed when your fog gets worse? Is it when you are rushed? Criticised? Trying to prove yourself? Sitting in a medical appointment where you sense you are not fully heard?

When I first began to see this pattern in clinic, I

had to confront something uncomfortable. I used to assume that if someone had brain fog, we needed to "improve" their cognition. Train it. Optimise it. Strengthen it.

But here is what experience has taught me... the brain follows safety, not effort.

When the nervous system feels guarded, energy is diverted. Focus narrows. Language falters. Memory slows. Not because you are incapable. But because you are conserving.

So what do you do with that?

You reduce demand.

Not dramatically. Not heroically. Quietly.

Standardise your meals. Eat similar foods at similar times. Boring? Perhaps. Stabilising? Absolutely. The fewer metabolic surprises your body has to manage, the less background noise your brain carries.

Reduce daily choices. Decision fatigue is real. I noticed this in my own life. When I simplified what I wore and ate during intense work periods, my mental bandwidth expanded. Small things matter.

Limit information intake. Do you really need another podcast? Another forum? Another article about symptoms? The truth is, constant input keeps the system on alert. Curate what enters your mind.

Single-task. One thing. Finish it. Then move on. Multitasking feels efficient, but it fragments attention and keeps the brain scanning.

Build predictable routines. Morning light. A regular wind-down. Repetition is not dullness. It is neurological reassurance.

And here is your quick win.

Choose one thing to stop deciding today.

Just one.

Perhaps dinner. Perhaps what you are wearing. Perhaps whether you will respond to that email. Remove the decision. Notice what happens in your body when something is already settled.

You may feel a small drop in tension. That is

cognitive load releasing.

There are common traps here.

Brain-training apps promise sharper thinking. Information overload masquerades as empowerment. Forcing focus feels disciplined.

But forcing is still pressure.

The truth is, you cannot bully your brain back into clarity.

When I have tried to push through my own mental fatigue—when I have told myself to "just concentrate harder"—it has always backfired. My body tightens. My recall worsens. The harder I try, the less fluid I become.

But when I reduce variables? When I stabilise routines? When I step out of environments where I feel subtly judged?

Clarity returns.

Not all at once. But steadily.

Your cognition is responsive. Not ruined.

When you feel believed, it strengthens. When your days become predictable, it settles. When you remove unnecessary decisions, it frees up energy.

Time and again, I see the same pattern... the fog lifts when the system no longer needs it.

You do not need to become sharper.

You need to become safer.

Your brain is not broken.

It is waiting for conditions that allow it to think clearly again.

Chapter Six - Rebuilding Trust - With Your Body and the Future

There is a moment that comes, often quietly, where something in you holds back.

Not from laziness.
Not from lack of will.

But because hope has asked too much of you before.

You have tried. Properly tried. Followed the plans. Paid for the programmes. Rearranged your days around protocols, appointments, new routines. You told yourself, *this time it will be different*. And when it wasn't, something in you became more careful.

The truth is... disappointment leaves an imprint.

You miss your old body. The one that did not need negotiation. The one that didn't require energy budgeting before a simple outing. You miss waking up with an assumption of capability, not a calculation of risk.

And here is the uncomfortable truth: it is not effort you fear.
It is being let down again.

Can you feel that distinction?

In my experience, when trust breaks with the body, it rarely collapses all at once. It thins out. Quietly. One cancelled plan. One flare after optimism. One professional dismissal that lands heavier than it should.

So now, when something improves, you don't celebrate. You monitor. You wait. You keep a layer of distance.

That is not negativity.
That is grief, expressed through caution.

You may remember the woman I introduced back in Chapter 3—the one living with persistent ulcers on her lower leg. Painful. Relentless. Her world had narrowed to dressings and careful movement. Progress was slow enough to almost disappear.

Then one morning, something shifted. The wound had begun to dry. A scab had formed.

Nothing dramatic. No announcement. Just a change in tissue.

She bent down and touched her leg for the first time in months. Not to manage it. Not to brace. Simply to feel it.

And in that moment, hope returned. Not as belief. Not as forced positivity. But as something quieter, more grounded.

Evidence.

The truth is... trust rebuilds through what the body demonstrates, not what the mind is told.

Not promises.
Not persuasion.
But proof.

A scab forming.
A slightly deeper sleep.
Less reactivity after a difficult day.

Small shifts your system recognises without needing to be convinced.

And yet, even when those shifts begin, many

people remain in management mode.

Energy is still rationed. Symptoms are still monitored. Plans are still made with an exit strategy. Life is lived as though the storm is still overhead—even when the weather has started to change.

Why does that happen?

Because vigilance once protected you.

What I have observed, time and again, is that the body becomes efficient at survival far quicker than it becomes comfortable with safety. Gearing up is fast. Standing down is slower.

I saw this very clearly in myself.

On my final day in a professional environment that had been out of alignment for longer than I care to admit, I joined a meeting already feeling the early signs of angioedema. The itching had started beneath the skin. A familiar signal.

In the past, I would have softened. Adjusted. Kept the peace at my own expense.

But that day, something was different.

I spoke directly. I asked for proper representation. And when it was clear that would not be met, I ended the call.

Within minutes, the itching stopped.

Not reduced. Not managed. Stopped.

No medication. No intervention. Just the absence of self-suppression.

When I stopped appeasing, my body stopped reacting.

The truth is... your body responds to what you *do,* not just what you intend.

You cannot rebuild trust while continuing to override yourself in subtle ways.

Without trust, progress slows. Even when capacity is returning. You can be improving physiologically and still living as though decline is inevitable.

And that is the real risk.

Not deterioration.
But remaining careful long after it is necessary.

So consider this, gently—where has your body already shifted, even slightly? What have you dismissed because it felt too small, too uncertain, too early to trust?

Because what becomes clear, over and over again, is that trust does not return in grand gestures. It returns in texture.

Softer mornings.
Quicker recovery.
A boundary held without consequence.
A wound drying.

You do not need to force confidence.

You need to notice what is already changing.

Your body has not been working against you. It has been protecting you. Sometimes intensely. Sometimes imperfectly. But always with the aim of keeping you going.

And when that level of protection is no longer required, it begins to ease.

Quietly. Gradually. Without announcement.

So perhaps the question is not, *can I believe again?*

Perhaps the question is, *can I let small evidence matter?*

That is where trust begins to rebuild.

The Body Reset Sequence™

Let me say something plainly.

You are not broken.

I know that sounds simple. Maybe even naïve. But stay with me.

When you've lived with symptoms for years—fatigue, palpitations, pain, fog, inflammation—you start to assume something inside you has permanently failed. Especially when you've done everything "right." The appointments. The prescriptions. The diets. The supplements. The therapy. The compliance.

And still... you wake up tired.

Still... you calculate your day like energy is a limited currency.
Still... you look functional on the outside and fragile on the inside.

Over years of observing this pattern, one thing has become consistently clear: most people are not dealing with a body that cannot heal. They are dealing with a body that does not feel safe enough to reorganise.

The truth is, healing is conditional.

And conditions can be changed.

That is where the Body Reset Sequence™ begins.

Not with force.
Not with belief.
With order.

Step 1 — Safety

Quiet the system input.

Let me ask you something.

When was the last time your body truly relaxed?

Not distracted.
Not medicated.
Not collapsed from exhaustion.

Actually relaxed.

Most people can't remember.

When you've been unwell for a long time, your nervous system lives on guard. Even good things feel like effort. Even hope feels risky.

I see this pattern constantly. Someone starts improving and immediately increases the load—more exercise, more commitments, more supplements, more "I'm back!"

And then the crash comes.

Have you noticed that cycle in yourself?

A good week. Then a collapse.

You call it bad luck. I call it overload.

The truth is, a dysregulated system interprets

change as threat. Even positive change.

When I first recognised this in my own clinical work, I had to face something uncomfortable. At times, the enthusiasm of recovery was actually destabilising people. More input. More stimulation. More striving.

What has become evident to me over time is this: safety is not emotional fluff. It is biological permission.

Safety means reducing sudden shifts. It means stopping the constant self-pressure to prove you're fine. It means not using every flicker of energy as a test of your worth.

Sometimes safety looks unremarkable.

Fewer variables.
Fewer experiments.
A steadier rhythm.

When I've seen someone pause at what I call the car park moment—that instant before pushing through, before filling the prescription that doesn't feel right, before overriding their body again—that is often the beginning.

A boundary.

A quiet decision: I am not adding more fire to a system already burning.

That is step one.

Step 2 — Signal Reduction

Remove the interference.

Now we go deeper.

If safety lowers the alarm, signal reduction clears the static.

Chronic illness often isn't a lack of effort. It's too much noise.

Too many inputs.
Too many protocols.
Too many opinions.
Too much self-monitoring.

Imagine trying to follow instructions in a room where ten radios are playing at once. You can still hear sound—but not direction.

The truth is, your body works through signals. Electrical. Chemical. Hormonal. Mechanical. When everything is flagged as urgent, nothing is prioritised properly.

This is why you can have “normal tests” and still feel dreadful.
This is why you can take the right medication and not respond.
This is why you can follow the textbook and still not stabilise.

I’ve watched people with significant medical interventions—stents, medications, careful management—continue to experience unpredictable tachycardia and exhaustion. Structure addressed. Regulation unresolved.

And here’s the hard truth: when you don’t feel believed, the noise increases.

When your carefully gathered report is dismissed.
When your lived experience is reduced to anxiety.
When you are told “everything looks fine” while your body is clearly not fine.

That rupture adds stress.

The truth is, you cannot regulate in a constant state of defence.

Signal reduction means asking a different question:

What is interfering with my system's ability to interpret information clearly?

It may be sleep disruption. Blood sugar swings. Boom-and-bust pacing. Constant symptom checking. Emotional hypervigilance. Endless protocol hopping.

And here's the part people resist: sometimes the most powerful intervention is subtraction.

When I've guided people to reduce inputs rather than add more, it can feel counterintuitive—almost like giving up.

But it isn't giving up.

It is making space.

A clearer way of putting it might be this: the system begins to function better when it is no longer overwhelmed by competing demands.

You are not doing less.

You are allowing clarity to return.

Step 3 — Cooperation

Gentle responsiveness returns.

Now something interesting happens.

When the alarm lowers and the noise reduces, your body starts responding differently.

Not dramatically.

Subtly.

This is cooperation.

And cooperation is fragile at first.

I often describe chronic illness as a workplace where every department has stopped trusting management. Hormones are doing one thing. Immune function is doing another. Cardiovascular regulation is improvising. Sleep is unreliable.

Everyone is in crisis mode.

The truth is, you cannot bully that system back into harmony.

You can threaten it.
You can escalate treatment.
You can warn of worst-case scenarios.

But fear does not create cooperation.

I've seen clients told, "If this doesn't improve, you'll be in a wheelchair." I understand the clinical intent. But physiologically? That lands as danger.

And danger shuts listening down.

Cooperation returns when your system no longer feels attacked.

You may notice small shifts:

You tolerate a walk without a surge in heart rate.
Your digestion steadies.
A stressful conversation doesn't cost you two days.
You wake one morning and don't immediately scan for symptoms.

Tiny things.

Do you dismiss them?

Most people do.

Because you've been disappointed before.

The truth is, cautious optimism is wise. Blind optimism isn't.

When I've worked with someone rebuilding trust, we don't celebrate prematurely. We observe. We gather data. We let the pattern prove itself.

What I have consistently seen is this: cooperation grows when you treat your body as intelligent, not defective.

You stop fighting it.

You start listening.

Step 4 — Capacity

Energy stabilises.

This is where life begins to expand again.

Not explosively.

Gradually.

Capacity isn't about having boundless energy. It's about predictability.

And if you have experienced what many of my clients have—waking already tired, scanning your body for symptoms, calculating every task before you do it—you will know how precious predictability is.

When I ask people what they want most, they rarely say "perfect health." They say, "I just want to know what I can rely on."

The truth is, capacity grows when your baseline steadies.

Your system isn't burning energy on constant threat detection. It isn't firefighting internal chaos. It has reserves again.

But here's the trap.

As soon as you feel better, you try to catch up.

You say yes to everything.
You restart the gym.

You take on extra work.
You test your limits.

Why?

Because you're afraid it won't last.

And when the relapse comes, it feels like betrayal.

The truth is, it wasn't betrayal. It was premature load.

When I've had to learn this lesson myself—and I have—I realised something humbling. Improvement is not an invitation to sprint. It is an invitation to stabilise.

Capacity grows under steady demand.

Not spikes.

If you respect that rhythm, energy becomes less volatile. Less fragile. More dependable.

And that changes how you see your future.

Step 5 — Exit Readiness

Management becomes unnecessary.

This step surprises people.

Because exit readiness isn't dramatic.

There's no fanfare. No declaration of cure.

It's quieter than that.

You realise you haven't thought about your symptoms all morning.
You travel without packing for catastrophe.
A bad night doesn't become a bad week.
You make plans without calculating the crash.

The truth is, you stop organising your life around avoidance.

That is freedom.

Not perfection. Freedom.

And something else shifts here too.

You re-enter medical conversations differently.

You are no longer pleading to be believed.

You are collaborating.

When I've seen this stage emerge, the person feels grounded. Not defensive. Not desperate. Just clear.

They know their baseline.
They recognise early overload.
They don't panic at normal fluctuation.

What becomes increasingly clear at this stage is this: when regulation returns, management stops being your identity.

You become a person again.

Not a case.
Not a syndrome.

A person.

Real-World Application — Cautious Trust

Let me show you what this looks like in real life.

Someone begins this process with very little

hope left. Not dramatic hopelessness. Quiet exhaustion.

They have tried everything. Spent money. Followed instructions. Joined communities that normalised suffering until it felt permanent.

So when improvement begins, they don't celebrate.

They watch.

Week one: standing at the kitchen counter a little longer without the heart racing.
Week two: the afternoon crash softens.
Week three: waking and, for a few seconds, forgetting to scan for symptoms.

That moment can feel surprising.

Have you ever had that? A small window where your body feels... neutral?

The instinct is to rush. To prove things are back to normal.

But something different happens.

There is a pause.

The pattern is remembered.

So instead of escalating, there is stabilising.

Instead of chasing certainty, there is quiet observation.

The truth is, trust rebuilds through repetition.

Not declarations.
Not affirmations.

Reliable evidence.

And over time—this is the part that matters—the body stops feeling like an adversary.

It begins to feel responsive.

That is trust.

Trust does not come back because you decide it should.
It returns when your body shows you something

different.

Small things. Subtle things. But real.

And in my experience... your system does not respond to motivation. It responds to evidence.

So we begin there.

Notice what works consistently

Not what worked once on a good day.
Not what worked because you were running on adrenaline.

What works again and again?

Ask yourself that honestly.

Is it eating at roughly the same times?
Going to bed before you are overtired?
Stopping work when you first feel the dip instead of pushing through?

The truth is, your nervous system trusts rhythm more than intensity.

When I stopped experimenting with myself

every week and instead repeated the same simple structure for a month, I noticed something uncomfortable at first.

Nothing dramatic happened.

But nothing dramatically fell apart either.

Stability is not exciting. It is healing.

Start writing things down. One page. One column. Title it: *What Actually Helps*. No theories. No hopes. Just observations.

You are gathering data, not chasing miracles.

Stop chasing fixes

This one can feel brutal.

Because searching feels active. Searching feels hopeful. Searching feels like you are doing something.

But the truth is, constant searching keeps your body on alert. It sends the signal that something is always wrong.

Have you noticed that?

Every new supplement. Every new protocol. Every new practitioner. A brief lift. Then uncertainty again.

What I've seen time and again is this... when you are always looking for the next fix, your system never settles long enough to recalibrate.

So try something brave.

Choose a window of time. Four weeks, perhaps. No new interventions unless medically essential. No radical eliminations. No dramatic additions.

Let the waters go still.

It may feel uncomfortable. You might worry you are missing something.

But you are not doing nothing.

You are observing.

And observation builds trust.

Honour small gains

This is harder than it sounds.

Because when you get a slightly better day, what do you want to do?

Use it.

Catch up. Prove something. Clean the house. Answer everything. Push.

I've done that. Many times.

And when I did, I paid for it.

The truth is, small gains are not invitations to sprint. They are signs that your system is stabilising.

If your energy lasts 20 minutes longer, protect it.
If your pain drops by two points, respect it.
If you sleep a little deeper, note it.

Over years of watching this pattern... the body learns safety through repetition, not celebration.

You do not need to announce improvement. You need to preserve it.

Reduce contingency planning

You have become very good at predicting disaster.

You scan for exits. You calculate how long you can last. You mentally rehearse what to say if you need to leave.

That skill protected you.

But here is the hard truth: constant anticipation of collapse keeps your nervous system braced.

When I realised how often I was planning for things to go wrong—even on calm days—I saw how much energy that forecasting consumed.

So experiment gently.

Choose one small activity this week where you do not rehearse the crash.

Not recklessly. Not foolishly. Just without running the full catastrophe script.

Go to the café without mapping the nearest toilet.
Attend the meeting without planning your apology.
Take the short walk without calculating the return route every five minutes.

Then observe.

Did the predicted disaster happen?

Sometimes it will. Often it will not.

Each time it does not, your system learns something new.

Allow cautious hope

Not grand hope. Not loud hope.

Cautious hope.

Hope that says, *Maybe this is not permanent.*

You may resist this. I understand that.

Because if you allow hope and it collapses, it hurts.

But the truth is, demanding certainty before you soften keeps you locked in vigilance.

You do not need guarantees.

You need possibility.

In practice, what becomes clear is this... healing often begins not when symptoms vanish, but when fear reduces by a fraction.

Let that be enough.

Common mistakes to watch for

You may demand certainty before you relax.
You may rush the moment you feel stronger.
You may compare yourself to who you were ten years ago and decide you have failed.

Please hear this clearly.

You are not rebuilding the past.

You are building capacity in the present.

Different body. Different season. Different wisdom.

When I stopped measuring myself against my former output and instead asked, *What is manageable now?* something shifted internally.

Pressure eased.

And, unexpectedly, capacity increased.

A simple daily practice

Before you sleep tonight, ask one question:

What did my body do right today?

Just one thing.

Did it regulate your temperature?
Digest a meal?
Recover from a spike faster than usual?
Hold you upright through a conversation?

Write it down.

This is not forced positivity. It is training perception.

Because the truth is, your body is doing thousands of things right every day—even in illness.

Trust does not rebuild through persuasion.

It rebuilds through accumulated evidence.

One steadier morning.
One boundary held.
One small gain protected.
One evening where you noticed what worked instead of what failed.

The future does not need to be guaranteed.

It only needs to remain open.

And for now, that openness is enough.

Trust does not come back in a grand gesture.
It comes back in inches.

You already know this. We have seen it through the stories earlier in this chapter. The drying wound. The Zoom call. Different contexts. Same principle.

What I have observed, time and again, is this: the body believes what it can measure.

Not what you hope.
Not what you affirm.
What it can physically experience.

Think about the woman with the ulcers we spoke about before. Months of open skin. Careful treatment. Endless patience. And then one small change — a scab forming at the edge. Nothing dramatic. No celebration. Just tissue doing something different.

She bent down and touched her leg.

That moment mattered.

The truth is, trust rebuilds through evidence. A scab. A calmer heartbeat. One afternoon without a crash. One meeting you leave without spiralling.

You may be waiting for certainty. But what if trust is simply repetition? What if it is your nervous system noticing, again and again, that today was slightly safer than yesterday?

It is not glamorous. It is not loud. It is biological.

And here is the harder truth: grief will sit beside you while this happens.

You will grieve the years lost.
You will grieve the strength you once had.
You may grieve the person you were before symptoms took over.

Does that mean you are going backwards?

No.

In my experience, grief and recovery are not opposites. They run in parallel. When the body feels safer, emotion thaws. When emotion thaws, grief surfaces. That is not failure. That is thawing tissue, thawing memory, thawing identity.

When I left a professional environment that had slowly eroded my alignment, my body told the story before I did. As I mentioned earlier, the angioedema began during a video meeting. The itching under the skin. The swelling trying to form.

I knew that pattern.

In the past, I would have softened my words. Stayed agreeable. Endured. But that day I didn't. I asked for proper representation. I named what wasn't working. And when it was clear nothing would change, I ended the call.

Within minutes, the itching stopped.

No ritual. No technique. Just alignment.

The truth is, when presence replaces appeasement, the body often stands down.

You have likely experienced your own version of this. A boundary held. A conversation left. A decision made. And suddenly, something settles.

Why?

Because the nervous system responds to safety, not performance.

What becomes clear over time is this: cooperation returns quietly. It does not ask for applause. It simply withdraws the alarm.

And this is why the exit from chronic illness is not a leap.

It is not one heroic act.
It is not one perfect protocol.
It is not a dramatic before-and-after.

It is a series of small, undeniable shifts.

You notice you are planning less around fear.
You notice a symptom does not escalate as it used to.
You notice you touch the place that once terrified you.

At first, these changes feel fragile. You do not trust them. That makes sense. You have been disappointed before.

But if the evidence keeps repeating, what happens then?

Trust begins to accumulate.

Like rings in a tree. Quiet. Structural. Invisible from the outside.

And one day you realise something subtle has changed in your language. You are no longer constantly "managing." You are observing. Adjusting. Participating.

The truth is, the exit is already underway long before you feel confident enough to name it.

You are not leaping out of illness.
You are walking out. Step by step. System by system.

And whether you fully believe it yet or not, this is the shift:

You are no longer organising your life around being unwell.

You are preparing to leave it behind.

Afterword

Leaving the Loop

When you began this book, you were not looking for inspiration.

You were looking for **relief that made sense**.

You were tired of being told your tests were normal while your life quietly narrowed. Tired of managing symptoms without understanding why they kept returning. Tired of doing everything "right" and feeling worse for the effort.

You may have arrived here sceptical—perhaps hopeful, but guarded. You had learned, through experience, not to trust promises easily. You had tried medicine. You had tried alternatives. You had tried explaining yourself, improving yourself, regulating yourself.

And somewhere along the way, you began to wonder whether the problem was *you*.

This book asked you to pause that assumption.

You learned, early on, that **normal results do not equal a regulated system**. That what you were experiencing was not invisible failure, but undetected dysregulation. You learned the difference between pathology and overload—and why fragmented care could never resolve a whole-system problem.

You stopped seeing yourself as a medical mystery or a difficult case.
You reclaimed dignity.

You then faced a harder truth: that trying harder was not helping—because effort itself was costing you more than it gave back. You learned to recognise borrowed energy, post-exertional crashes, and the subtle ways self-management drains capacity. You were given permission—perhaps for the first time—to subtract rather than optimise.

You learned why treatments that *should* have worked didn't. Not because your body was resistant, broken, or uncooperative—but because **receptivity had been lost**. Through Signal Reception Theory™, you learned to recognise non-response as a safety signal rather than a verdict. You learned when pausing is not giving up—but restoring conditions for response.

You learned something else that may have surprised you: that talking—however well-intentioned—can sometimes make the body worse. That insight without safety is not neutral. That the nervous system must be stabilised before it can tolerate reflection. You learned that healing does not require reliving, narrating, or explaining yourself again.

You learned that your brain is not broken. That fog is not decline, but overload. That clarity returns not through training or effort, but through predictability, reduced input, and restored regulation.

And finally, you learned that the loss of trust you carried—toward medicine, alternatives, and your own body—was not weakness. It was a rational response to repeated non-response. You learned how trust returns: not through hope or pressure, but through small, consistent signals of cooperation.

If nothing else, you leave this book knowing this:

Your body was not failing you.
It was protecting itself the only way it could.

And now, conditions have changed.

KEY TAKEAWAYS SUMMARY

Return to these principles whenever you feel pulled back into urgency or self-doubt:

- **Normal results do not equal normal regulation.**
Dysregulation exists long before damage appears.

- **Effort is not neutral.**
In depleted systems, trying harder accelerates collapse.

- **Receptivity precedes response.**
A body must be able to receive before it can improve.

- **Timing matters more than dosage.**
When input arrives too early, even help becomes noise.

- **Non-response is a safety signal, not resistance.**

Pausing can restore capacity faster than persisting.

- **Insight without safety destabilises the body.**

Regulation must come before reflection.

- **Brain fog reflects overload, not decline.**

Clarity returns through subtraction and predictability.

- **Trust is rebuilt physiologically, not emotionally.**

Small, reliable improvements matter more than belief.

- **Management is not recovery.**

Regulation replaces vigilance when conditions allow.

These are not motivational ideas.
They are organising principles.
You can return to them whenever the ground feels unsteady.

WHAT'S NEXT: A QUIET QUESTION

At this point, something subtle has likely shifted.

Your system is quieter.
Your responses are more predictable.
Your body is no longer fighting everything you offer it.

And a new question may be forming—not urgently, but naturally:

If force, effort, and belief weren't required... what actually allowed regulation to return?

That question marks the transition from *exit* to *understanding*.

The Chronic Illness Exit Plan focused on **removal**—quieting the system so cooperation could re-emerge. It showed you what to stop doing so your body could stabilise.

The next book in this series, **Energy Without Belief**, begins where this one ends.

It explains what is now accessible.

Without spiritual language.
Without blind faith.
Without asking you to adopt a philosophy.

Energy Without Belief introduces energy as **function**—as biological signalling, resonance, feedback, and coherence operating below thought and belief. It explains why gentle regulation succeeds where force fails, and why sceptical systems often respond best.

If this book helped you exit the loop, the next one helps you **understand the layer of regulation that is now active**—so you can work with it intelligently, safely, and without abandoning scientific restraint.

There is no rush.

But there is a next step, when you're ready.

If this book has been helpful, here are a few gentle ways to continue:

1. Stay Connected

You can join the email list on www.thestreetholistics.com for occasional resources—simple templates, clarifying diagrams, and updates related to the Chronic Illness Exit Plan™. No urgency. No overwhelm. Just practical support when it's useful.

2. Leave a Review

If this book helped you see your body differently, a brief review helps others like you find it. Quiet, honest reflections matter more than praise.

3. Continue with Book 2

If you're ready to understand what's now happening beneath the surface, *Energy Without Belief* is the natural next step in this journey.

You were never meant to cope forever.

You were meant to understand enough to step out of the loop—and let your body do what it was trying to do all along.

This is not the end.

It is a quieter beginning.

About the Author

Dr. June Williams writes for those who have reached the edge of conventional answers—and sense, quietly but unmistakably, that something vital has been overlooked.

With a background in biology and a Doctorate in Medical Ethics, she spent over three decades within clinical research. Yet it was not what medicine could explain that shaped her work—it was what it could not.

Her approach reframes chronic illness not as failure, but as a form of intelligent response—an accumulation of overload, interference, and disrupted communication within the body's systems.

Through her work, she offers a different way forward. One that does not rely on force, belief, or endless intervention—but on restoring the conditions in which the body can begin to regulate again.

Drawing on Bioresonance, integrative hypnotherapy, the Metamorphic Technique, and Systemic Constellations, she has developed a practical, non-talking framework designed to help individuals step out of chronic patterns and into measurable change.

The Chronic Illness Exit Plan is not another method to manage symptoms. It is an invitation to leave the loop entirely.

Learn more at: www.thestreetholistics.com

The Books in the Series

1. *The Chronic Illness Exit Plan*
A clear starting point when nothing has worked—and no one has given you answers.

2. *Energy Without Belief*
A scientific introduction to subtle regulation, explained without spirituality or hype.

3. *Bioresonance Explained for Real People*
A practical, honest guide to what Bioresonance is—and what it is not.

4. *Emotional Healing Without Reliving Trauma*
How to resolve emotional load without talking therapy or re-traumatisation.

5. *The Exit Is Not the End*
How to stabilise, rebuild, and live well after chronic illness.